Graham Harvey won the BP Natural Book Prize for *The Killing of the Countryside* in 1997. He is an agriculture graduate and has written on rural issues for *New Scientist, Private Eye, The Sunday Times* and the *Daily Mail*. A former script writer of *The Archers*, he is currently the programme's Agricultural Story Editor.

Praise for *The Killing of the Countryside*

'A modern *Grapes of Wrath* . . . I have seldom read a more meticulous or devastating case for the prosecution.'
Simon Jenkins, The Times

Praise for *The Forgiveness of Nature*

'Consistently gripping . . . A terrific book.'   *Daily Mail*

Acknowledgements

Special thanks to Margaret Adams, Jim and Kay Barnard, Malcolm Bole, Brian Castle, Mark Draper, Sally Fallon, Neil Hopkin, Danny Goodwin Jones, Martin Lane, David Marsh, Robert Plumb, John Reeves, Lyn Searby, David Thomas, Richard Vincent, Peter Wallace, David Henry Wilson, Walter Yellowlees and, not least, my wife Annie, whose support and encouragement has been, as always, unstinting.

Other books by Graham Harvey

The Killing of the Countryside

We Want Real Food

Why our food is deficient in minerals and nutrients – and what we can do about it

Graham Harvey

CONSTABLE • LONDON

Constable & Robinson Ltd
3 The Lanchesters
162 Fulham Palace Road
London W6 9ER
www.constablerobinson.com

First published in the UK by Constable,
an imprint of Constable & Robinson Ltd, 2006

A copy of the British Library Cataloguing in
Publication Data is available from the British Library.

ISBN-10: 1-84529-267-7
ISBN-13: 978-1-84529-267-6

Printed and bound in the EU

1 3 5 7 9 10 8 6 4 2

Contents

1
The Nature of Sweetness

It started with a bunch of organic bananas. I bought them in a wholefood shop. They hadn't looked particularly promising – a sort of washed out grey in colour, but I felt sure they'd ripen once I got them home.

A week later they were starting to go soft, though the skin had turned even greyer. I peeled one and took a bite. It wasn't that it tasted bad. Quite the opposite. There was no discernible taste of any kind. Not so much as the merest hint of sweetness. I might as well have been eating damp cardboard.

This came as something of a shock. If it had been the usual chemically-grown stuff I'd have understood. No one expects the economy end of the fresh produce market to taste of anything much these days, but we're talking organic here. These bananas had been grown without any chemical sprays, and nourished with barrow-loads of good, old-fashioned compost – or so I imagined. They *ought* to have been full of flavour.

Then again, maybe I shouldn't have been that surprised. To be honest, I'd experienced tasteless organic produce before – carrots that hardly registered on the taste buds; apples with all the sweetness and flavour of household soap.

I used to believe it didn't matter much. Why worry about the taste, I thought, so long as they're doing you good. I know better these days.

As a kid I remember being intrigued by the picture on the tin of Lyle's Golden Syrup. It shows a dead lion with a swarm of bees coming out. The proverb that goes with it is a bit of a mystery too: 'Out of the strong came forth sweetness.'

The picture's still there on the Golden Syrup tin – I checked in my local superstore. It's from the Bible story of Samson. While travelling to Timnah, Samson is attacked by a young lion. He kills it with his bare hands. On the return journey he notices that the carcass has been occupied by the bees. So he scoops out the honey to sustain him on his journey.

Ironically, it was nineteenth-century sugar refiners like Abram Lyle, of Lyle's Golden Syrup, who made it possible to put a sweet taste in junk foods. Before they started turning out their deadly white crystals, sweetness had long been associated with strength and vitality.

In nature, sweetness is often linked to rich sources of essential trace elements, such as zinc, magnesium, copper and boron. Sweet-tasting natural foods like ripe fruits, berries and honey contain minerals as well as sugars. For early man – the hunter-gatherer – there was an evolutionary advantage in developing a sweet tooth. It was a means of selecting the ripest fruits, which would be at their most nutritious.

But fresh foods no longer taste sweet. Many are deliberately harvested whilst under-ripe, to lessen damage in transport and extend shelf life. Also, they've been robbed of many of the trace elements they once contained although this is disputed by some food scientists (see page 53). A revolution in the way they're grown has taken away the very nutrients that once promoted good health. Our staple foods have been 'dumbed down'. As a result, Britain – like other industrial countries – is suffering a tidal wave of sickness.

Degenerative conditions, such as heart disease, arthritis, diabetes and asthma, are reaching epidemic proportions. No fewer than one in three of us will be struck down with cancer at some stage in our lives. Mental illness, too, is rife – everything from depression to dementia.

Could food really be responsible for the health catastrophe that has overtaken the western world? It seems scarcely credible. Yet the fact remains that our basic foods have been changed. They are now subtly different from those eaten by human beings through all of history.

Britain – like other western countries – is fifty years into a mass experiment in human nutrition. We're all eating basic foods that have been stripped of the antioxidants, trace elements and essential fatty acids that once promoted good health. Is it any wonder that our body maintenance systems are breaking down in middle age or earlier?

Nitrogen compounds – the products of a worldwide chemical industry – are the powerhouse that drives modern farming. It's those small, white pellets – prills, as the manufacturers call them – that have degraded our everyday foods and led to the upsurge in ill-health.

Nitrogen fertilizers weaken plants by stimulating excess growth of sappy tissue with thin cell walls. Crops grown this way are more prone to disease, which is why they need constant spraying with chemicals to keep them standing. And when fed to livestock, they are unlikely to promote health in the animals: hence the need for routine antibiotics. So it's no real surprise that such crops are no better for people.

There was a time when the British were rather good at farming. As far back as Roman times, these islands off the north-west coast of Europe were regularly exporting wheat back to the mainland. They had been blessed with deep, fertile soils – a legacy of the post-glacial forest – and a mild, moist climate that was superb for growing a wide range of crops.

In the late eighteenth century, the island farmers developed a revolutionary cropping system that practically doubled the output of food. It was a clever way of alternating cereals with livestock-feeding crops, especially root crops and clover, which adds nitrogen to the soil naturally.

Admittedly, it wasn't an entirely original idea. The farmers of Flanders had been doing something similar for centuries.

Some of the best vegetables I ever tasted were grown by a runaway monk. For twenty years he had lived a life of prayerful contemplation. Then out of the blue he fell in love with a travelling piano tuner. And suddenly his world was on its head.

Today, the two of them share a small Dorset cottage with a five-acre paddock attached. While she journeys to the distant parts of Wessex tuning up neglected Steinways, he pours his new-found happiness into the small market garden he is creating on his rich, dark soil.

So fertile and productive are his deep beds that his crops seem to come springing out of them like grass after rain in an arid valley.

I met Jonno by pure chance, while driving down his quiet lane. Lashed to a tree was his hand-painted sign with the day's offerings chalked on it. That's about the only advertising he does.

But when I tried the carrots and plump, ripe tomatoes, I was hooked. Nowadays I call in whenever I'm that way. I buy anything that's going – a bundle of asparagus or a bag of rich, dark cherries; a punnet of sweet strawberries or a dozen mahogany brown eggs from his high-stepping Marans. All are so filled with flavour that you wonder whether the supermarket versions can be the same foods.

Occasionally, in summer there might even be a pack of soft yellow butter, the sort you never see in stores. Jonno has a house cow – a quiet, doe-eyed Jersey of advancing age. She was on her fifth calf when he bought her and there have been four more since. She walks placidly round her paddock, more often than not with a calf in tow.

Her eye is bright; her dark tan coat gleams in the sunlight. She has the quiet confidence of one who is comfortable in the company of humans.

Next door to the little holding is a commercial dairy farm. There must be at least two hundred in the herd, all high-yielding black-and-white Holsteins. When they're grazing the field the other side of Jonno's hedge, it's like having an invading army camped outside. In a day or two they'll have the turf stripped bare and be waiting at the gate baying for fresh pasture.

We stand and watch as they tear at the grass, compelled to fill the enormous udders that science and the cattle breeders have lumbered them with. Though few are over five years old, their skin hangs loose from the bones. Everything has been sacrificed to the white liquid and the instinct to feed offspring they're never allowed to keep.

These are the beasts that fill our daily milk cartons and yogurt pots. This is the kind of herd that stocks the supermarket chill cabinets. They're also the beasts that gave the world mad cow disease and the biggest outbreak of foot-and-mouth disease for decades.

Disease is the shadow that hangs permanently over herds like this. So unhealthy and overworked are the cows that they're worn out after three or four years' milking. They only survive as long as they do because they're routinely dosed with antibiotics.

Like modern-day vegetables, the forage crops grown for livestock have been robbed of the minerals and nutrients the animals need to stay healthy. And the root cause of the sickness – in humans as in farm animals – is a group of chemicals that farmers have come to rely on for almost everything they produce.

Half a dozen times during the growing season, Jonno's dairy-farming neighbour drives his tractor to and fro across his pasture fields, sowing a mass of small, white pellets. They contain compounds of nitrogen in one form or another – in Britain it's most likely to be ammonium nitrate.

But British farmers were smart enough to pick it up and apply it on a grand scale. That's how they were able to feed the nation during the Industrial Revolution, a time of unprecedented population growth.

In Victorian times, British farming was known and admired across the world. Our great breeds of cattle – the Hereford, the Shorthorn, the North Devon, the Aberdeen Angus, the Sussex, the Welsh Black and the Ayrshire – were sought after everywhere. For the best part of a century, Britain could justly claim to be stud farm to the world.

Now nobody wants our cattle. The land of legendary farmers is better known today as the birthplace of mad cow disease – a country of sickness and fear. The defining image of British agriculture is no longer the magnificent Hereford bull, once famed the world over. It is the pyre of burning cattle carcasses, fiery beacon of the foot-and-mouth crisis of 2001.

Feeding people well ought to be easy by now. After all, we've been at it long enough. Farming of one sort or another has been around for 12,000 years.

The principles of sound agriculture hardly change from generation to generation. Why should they? The human body has scarcely altered since the Stone Age. The foods required to keep it in good working order are no different from those of the hunter-gatherers, or the first farmers as they planted their primitive cereals in a scratched-out seedbed.

The only requirement for wholesome, nutrient-rich crops is a fertile soil. It's the same for livestock. When it comes to raising cattle for healthy beef or dairy products, all you need is a field or two of good grassland – grown on a fertile soil. And this is the very thing that chemical fertilizers have destroyed.

Whenever I take the train north, I pass a series of intensive vegetable fields strung out alongside the railway. The sight of this sad ground invariably fills me with gloom. In the summer months it's mostly planted up with salads or veg, laser-straight lines of cabbages, carrots or iceberg lettuce. From the train you can see the tramlines, the spaced tractor wheel marks that show the pesticide sprayer is frequently taken through the crop.

In the winter the ground is bare. There's not a weed to be seen. When the weather's wet, great pools of water lie on the surface unable to drain away. The bare ground in between has crusted over, making it impossible for air to penetrate into the soil spaces and supply the myriad life forms that could give the land 'heart' and help grow healthy plants.

Even from the train you can see this land is sick. So drenched has it been in chemical sprays and fertilizers that its normal function has virtually broken down. The robust crumb structure, which allows water and air to pass through the top layers, has disappeared. Beneficial organisms like earthworms will have suffocated – to thrive they need well-aerated soils with open channels and pore space.[1] Deep below the surface, processes of putrefaction will be taking place. The only way vegetable plants can be induced to grow here is with constant spraying with pesticides, otherwise they will inevitably succumb to disease.

Who will buy these vegetables, I wonder. They'll have been washed and packed for a supermarket somewhere. Perhaps it'll be some harassed young mum keen to do the best she can for her uninterested youngsters. She'll cajole them into trying a carrot or a floret or two of broccoli with their chicken dinosaurs. It'll do them good, she'll promise.

But she'll be wrong. There'll be precious little in those vegetables to help her kids grow up strong and healthy. Judging from the abused and miserable soil that grew them, it's hard to imagine they'll produce any sort of nourishment. The tragedy is that with a season or two of care and attention, those fields beside the railway tracks could begin growing the sort of food that would make her kids as strong as lions.

Is it any wonder that today's youngsters have little interest in fresh foods? The desire for sweetness is instinctive. In evolutionary terms, it directed the early hominid towards ripe fruits and vegetables, and away from poisonous plants that mostly tasted bitter.[2] Organic food offers no cast-iron guarantee of good nutrition. As the organic market expands, more crops are grown on land 'converted' after decades of chemical farming. Even under the new rules, there's no guarantee they'll be packed with the minerals and vitamins needed for good health.

Today the fields around us are filled with fantastic machines. There are tractors big enough to develop 500 horsepower at the flick of a switch. Modern forage harvesters can chomp their way through a field full of shoulder-high maize in less

Robert Plumb (see also page 177) is a soil doctor. His mission is to revitalize sick and ailing farmland, ruined by years of assault by chemical fertilizers. He started his career in the fertilizer business. For a time he ran his own 'blending' company, supplying nitrates and other chemical fertilizers to farmers.

Twenty years on, he's had a change of heart. He's convinced the constant use of chemicals has brought many soils to the verge of collapse, threatening public health. His company – Independent Soil Services – now advises worried farmers on how best to restore their damaged fields to health. That's the only way they can be made to grow good food again.

I met up with Plumb in a potato field in the Welsh Marches. The crop looked dense and green in the bright sunshine of an August morning. There was no sign of blight, the great scourge of potatoes, which had been the cause of the Irish famine. I assumed the field had been sprayed with fungicide, a precautionary measure taken by most non-organic growers to protect their investment.

But the crop hadn't been sprayed, Plumb assured me. There was no need. It stayed healthy because it was growing on a fertile soil.

Four years earlier it was a different story. A crop like this would have been impossible to grow, Plumb explained. The land had been so damaged by endless applications of nitrogen fertilizer, its structure had completely broken down.

With yields plummeting, the desperate farmer had sought specialist help. Plumb prescribed soil supplements to replace depleted minerals, particularly calcium. He also recommended organic compounds to re-invigorate the teeming mass of soil micro-organisms, which are the key to soil fertility.

Today the farmer has cut back dramatically on chemical sprays and fertilizers. At the same time he is growing better crops than for years.

I walked with Plumb into the potatoes for a closer look. An hour earlier there had been a heavy shower, and our trousers were quickly drenched. Even so, our boots remained remarkably free of mud, as Plumb was keen to point out.

'If we'd walked across this field a couple of years back,' he told me, 'we'd be carrying half a stone of soil on our boots by now. The soil structure was shot to hell. Even after a light shower you'd get pools of standing water. The ground was so compacted it couldn't drain away.

'Now there's a structure to the soil. There are plenty of air spaces, so the water can drain away. This means the plant roots can reach down to get the nutrients they need. This land is alive again. For the first time in years it's producing good, healthy food.'

To prove it, he gave me a raw potato to try. He took out a small garden trowel and dug up a single plant. The root held half a dozen or so serious-sized potatoes, plus a handful of tiddlers. Selecting one of the larger ones, he scraped away the dirt with the trowel. Then with his penknife he cut out a small square of the hard, white flesh. 'You try this,' he said with a smile.

I didn't relish it. Potato plants belong to the same family as the deadly nightshade. Because of their payload of toxic alkaloids, it's one of the few vegetables that's better for you cooked. But in the interests of research I thought I'd give it a go.

I bit into it. I'd been expecting the taste to be bland. Instead the overriding sensation was one of incredible sweetness. It was as if I'd bitten into a ripe dessert apple.

'That's what you get with a crop that's well-nourished,' said Plumb. 'The sweet taste tells you it's got a high mineral content. So it'll do you a lot more good than the average supermarket spud.'

time than it took a French peasant farmer thirty years ago to load up a single hay trailer.

Combine harvesters are now so smart that they can monitor their precise geographical position by satellite as they move through the crop, then record the grain yield of every square yard in a field the size of Heathrow Airport. But what use is this technology when it gathers second-rate foods from land that's worn out?

There's no machine yet that can add an extra microgram of iron to a wheat grain – no machine that'll boost the level of cancer-fighting vitamins in cows' milk. The only useful measure of a farming system is how well it feeds the people. On this basis, the new agricultural revolution – and the nitrogen fertilizers that power it – have been an unmitigated disaster.

Britain is now overwhelmingly an urban nation. Even so, you don't have to look far back in the histories of most families to find a link with the land.

I once spent fruitless hours searching through the 1881 census records, thankfully available on CD-ROM. I was trying to track down my great-grandfather, who I knew to have been a farmworker in north Berkshire.

For some reason I drew a blank. The name I'd been looking for didn't appear. But as I scrolled through the pages I was amazed at the number of men who – at a time of rapid industrialization – still entered their occupation as 'farm labourer'. Many would have been direct descendants of families who had milked their own cows and raised their own sheep and pigs until their land rights were snatched from them in the enclosures, the process through which common land was almost completely transferred into private ownership during the second half of the eighteenth and early nineteenth centuries.

Napoleon famously described the English as a nation of shopkeepers. But long before we became shopkeepers, we were a nation of small farmers. For the sake of our health it may be time to renew that acquaintance with the land.

Since Britain joined the European Community in 1973, we, the people, have paid out more than a hundred billion pounds in farm subsidies. The taxpayers have effectively bought and paid for the farmland on these islands. In return they should expect to eat well.

This is the story of a national treasure lost; a tale of paradise sprayed, poisoned and impoverished. It's also the story of how ridiculously easy it would be to get it back.

The American agrarian writer Gene Logsdon has a theory that sometime in the not-too-distant future, the food we eat will come from gardens rather than what we now call farms.[3] It's a fanciful notion, he admits. But no more fanciful than the idea that we can be fed by agribusiness companies like Monsanto and Cargill.

Even now, millions of people in Asia live well from the production of farms that are scarcely bigger than large gardens. While a mechanic building a car in his own garage can't compete with Ford or Honda, there's no agribusiness company on Earth that can grow a carrot cheaper or better than the backyard gardener.

For years Britain's farmland has been driven relentlessly to produce heavier crops at ever-lower cost. Now it's time to put it to a new purpose – restoring the people of these islands to health and happiness.

2
Minerals and Quarry Dust

One of the most remarkable studies, on the link between food and health, was carried out by an American dentist who is now hardly remembered.

In the early years of the twentieth century, Weston A. Price ran a thriving dental practice in the industrial city of Cleveland, Ohio. Then in the early 1930s he gave it all up. He and his wife set out on a series of epic journeys to some of the most remote places on the planet.

Price's idea was to visit peoples untouched by 'civilization' – peoples reputed to display remarkable health, and to enjoy long lives, untroubled by sickness and disease. He wanted to find out whether the stories were true. And if they were, he wanted to know what foods these peoples ate.

He published his exhaustive findings in 1939.[1] But in those tumultuous times no one took a great deal of notice, either in America or in Britain. This was a tragedy. Had they done so they might have spared both countries a catastrophic decline into obesity and ill health.

To live long and healthy lives, Price discovered, human beings needed the natural foods of the countryside, including animal products with their full complement of saturated fats.

These are not the kinds of foods that now cram the shelves of every neighbourhood supermarket. Nor are they the foods that pour from today's mechanized, chemically-driven agriculture.

In the 1930s, the American dentist Weston Price visited a secluded valley high in the Swiss Alps. Until the building of an eleven-mile-long railway tunnel a few years earlier, the Loetschental Valley in the Bernese Oberland had been virtually isolated from the outside world. There Price was astonished to find children tough enough to walk barefoot in freezing mountain streams without ill effects. These children seldom caught colds, and infections were virtually unknown. No case of tuberculosis (TB) had ever been seen among the valley community, though the people had been exposed to the bacillus. The children's teeth and gums were in perfect condition, Price discovered, with no sign of dental decay.

The people of this Swiss valley lived mainly on unpasteurized milk and dairy products from their own cows, which grazed on the steep mountain pastures.

They're foods that used to come from traditional farms of the sort western countries have done their best to eliminate.

By the time Price embarked on his travels, he had reached the very pinnacle of his profession. He had taught at American dental schools, written textbooks, and directed a classic study on the role of root canals in causing disease.[2] But his overriding interest was in nutrition and its effect on human health.

At that time, the people of Cleveland were abandoning their traditional diets in favour of the new, manufactured foods – white bread, margarine, pasteurized milk, and refined white sugar. Price saw the results daily in his surgery. Most of his adult patients had rampant tooth decay, often accompanied by degenerative diseases such as arthritis, osteoporosis and diabetes and by chronic fatigue.

The health of younger patients was even more worrying. Their teeth were often crowded and crooked. Many had facial deformities, such as 'overbites' and narrow, pinched faces with no well-defined cheekbones. The same children frequently

On the Isle of Lewis, off the north-west coast of Scotland, Price saw that the local people ate no dairy products at all. They lived mainly on cod and other seafoods, especially shellfish. These were supplemented with oatmeal. On the thin island soils, oats were the only grain that could be grown. A prized local dish – considered especially beneficial for growing children and pregnant women – was cod's head stuffed with oats and mashed fish liver.

suffered from other health complaints with names that sound all too familiar today – allergies, recurring infections, anaemia, asthma and behavioural difficulties. All these had been rare when Price had started in practice around the turn of the century.

One of the more serious infectious diseases of the day was TB, widely known as the 'White Scourge'. Price observed that children were increasingly afflicted by the disease. And among the most vulnerable youngsters were those with bad teeth. That's when he hit on the idea of travelling to places not yet 'touched' by civilization – journeys of discovery that were to preoccupy him for the next ten years.

Price and his wife visited tribes of hunter-gatherers in northern Canada, the Florida Everglades, the Amazon rainforest and Australia. These people consumed game meats of all types, especially offals. But they supplemented them with a variety of whole grains, vegetables and fruits.

Price also visited an Inuit (Eskimo) people, whose diet was almost wholly made up of animal products. These included fish, walrus, seal and other marine mammals. During the brief summer months the people would gather nuts, berries and a few grasses. These provided small diversions in a diet made up overwhelmingly of animal products, including large amounts of blubber (the fat of sea mammals).

In all corners of the world, Price found these remote peoples to be in perfect health. The foods they ate were, without exception, natural. There were no preservatives, colourings or additives; no refined oils or hydrogenated fats; no processed foods such as white flour or skimmed milk. Nor was there added sugar, though a number of peoples ate naturally sweet foods such as honey or maple syrup. All the foods were grown or raised on fertile soils, uncontaminated by pesticides or chemical fertilizers. Milk and dairy products were always consumed in their raw or unpasteurized state.

> Of the African peoples he visited, Price found the Dinkas of Sudan to be the most healthy. They ate a combination of fermented grains and fish, together with small amounts of red meat, vegetables and fruit. By contrast, cattle-herding tribes like the Masai ate no plants at all. They lived exclusively on beef, raw milk, offal meats, and – in times of drought – cattle blood.

Wherever he went, Price took photographs of the locals. By the time he'd finished his journeys, he had amassed no fewer than 18,000 photos. Some were later published in his classic book, *Nutrition and Physical Degeneration*. Today it serves as a remarkable social record of healthy, well-nourished people, with broad facial structures which allowed full development of the dental arch.

Nutrition researcher Sally Fallon – founder of the Weston A. Price Foundation in Washington – says of the book:

No one can look at the handsome photographs of so-called primitive people – faces that are broad, well-formed and noble – without realizing that there's something very wrong with the development of modern children.

In every isolated region he visited, Price found tribes or villages where virtually every individual exhibited genuine physical perfection. In such groups tooth decay was rare, and dental crowding and occlusions – the kind of problems that keep American orthodontists in yachts and vacation homes – were non-existent.

Price took photograph after photograph of beautiful smiles, and noted that the natives were invariably cheerful and optimistic. Such people were characterized by 'splendid physical development' and an almost complete absence of disease, even those living in physical environments that were extremely harsh.

As well as taking photographs, Price collected samples of local food wherever he travelled. Carefully preserving them, he brought them back to Cleveland. He wanted to find out whether such diverse natural diets had any common attributes that might account for the robust good health of those remote peoples.

In his laboratory he made detailed analyses of each sample, calculating its total complement of nutrients. From the full set of figures, he was able to calculate the nutrient intake of each community. The results amazed him. They showed that these health-giving diets contained at least four times the level of minerals and water-soluble vitamins – vitamins C and B-complex – than the average American diet of his day. And they contained no less than ten times the levels of fat-soluble vitamins, including vitamins A and D, together with a new nutrient he called 'activator X'.

Price considered these fat-soluble vitamins to be the key component of healthy diets. He called them 'activators' (or 'catalysts'), because the assimilation of all other nutrients in the diet – protein, minerals and water-soluble vitamins – depended on them. Price wrote:

> It is possible to starve for minerals that are abundant in the foods eaten because they cannot be utilized without an adequate quantity of the fat-soluble activators. The amounts [of nutrients] utilized depend directly on the presence of other substances, particularly the fat-soluble vitamins. It is at this point probably that the greatest

breakdown in our modern diet takes place, namely in the ingestion and utilization of adequate amounts of the special activating substances, including the vitamins, needed for rendering the minerals in the food available to the human system.

Price's 'activator X', a powerful catalyst to mineral absorption, occurred in foods considered valuable in many primitive societies: liver and other offal meats, fish liver oils, fish eggs and butter from cows grazing on rapidly-growing spring and autumn grass. These vital foods are mostly missing from the modern British diet. At a time when many of these foods have fallen from favour, the toll of degenerative diseases has risen inexorably.

Here was the reason for the legendary health and stamina of these remote peoples. Their staple foods – whether from the sea or from the land – were highly-mineralized and rich in antioxidants. And here was the reason for the worsening health in Price's city of Cleveland. The people's diets had been debased by the substitution of industrial foods for the natural foods of the countryside. And in the 60 years or so since, the situation has grown steadily worse.

Today's fresh produce has little in common with the nutrient-rich foods of pre-industrial societies. Years of chemical farming and soil mismanagement have robbed them of health-giving minerals and antioxidants. In the fresh produce sections of every neighbourhood supermarket, the shelves are packed with fruits and vegetables from around the globe. All are bright and colourful. The choice seems bewildering.

'Counts towards your five-a-day,' say the shelf labels, reinforcing the campaign to boost consumption of healthy foods. But at the heart of the display is a deception. However colourful they may look, few of these foods have the power to protect against illness. Their nutritive qualities have eroded away like the fertility of the soils that grew them. Today's fresh produce is all show and precious little substance.

Professor A. F. W. Brix was a nineteenth-century German chemist who will be forever revered by the world's winemakers.[3] It was Brix who devised a way of measuring the quality of grape juice using a hydrometer – an instrument that measures the density of liquids. His ingenious device enabled Europe's winemakers to assess the potential of a grape juice before going to the expense of fermenting and bottling it.

Today, the chemist's name is used as a measure of the quality of fresh produce. Strictly speaking, the 'Brix' number of a plant juice refers to its concentration of sugars, but American farm and health consultant Dr Carey A. Reams believed that this was itself linked to mineral content. In fact, the level of sugars correlated with a range of valuable materials, including amino acids, proteins and phytonutrients, so the Brix number was a good guide to food quality.

For example, a sour-tasting grape grown on an exhausted and over-worked soil is likely to give a Brix reading of 8 or less. But a full-flavoured grape grown on rich, fertile soil will give a reading of 24 or even higher. And what's true of grapes applies equally to other food plants. A Brix number is a measure of the real food value of the fresh produce in modern supermarkets.

There are two easy ways to measure the nutrient content of fresh foods. First you can taste them. Foods that seem bland and flavourless are almost certain to be low in essential minerals. Plants produce thousands of compounds that aren't essential for the vital life processes of the cell, but which give each plant species its own unique characteristics. It's these 'secondary metabolites' that give colour and fragrance to flowers, for example. They're also responsible for the tastes and textures of fruit and vegetables.

Minerals are essential for the cell processes that produce this battery of chemical compounds, so it's not surprising that fresh foods, which have strong flavours and fragrances, should be well-endowed with essential minerals. But for people who

My hand-held Brix refractometer arrived by post in a neat package bearing the name of the supply company in San Pedro, California. It had cost me about £35. Both my wife and I reckoned it was a small price to pay for the means to establish the quality of our foods.

The device looks a bit like a short telescope. At one end there's an eyepiece, at the other a small prism. It measures the quality of a plant juice by the degree light is bent – or refracted – when passing through it. The more dense the liquid, the more the light is refracted.

Thankfully, it's easy to use. First you have to extract a few drops of juice from the item under test. I did this by crushing a piece of apple in a standard garlic press. Then with a glass eye dropper, you have to transfer a drop or two on to the prism, and flatten it with the glass cover-plate. After that it's simply a matter of looking through the eyepiece and reading off the Brix number from a calibrated scale.

don't quite trust their taste buds, there's a second, less subjective way to tell if a food's any good or not. It's called the Brix refractometer, widely used by supermarkets to find out when fruit is ripe enough to be picked.

Using the Brix refractometer to first measure the quality of a home-grown apple, I then set out to test the integrity of our local supermarkets. In nearby Taunton I visited the three biggest stores – Tesco, Sainsbury's and Morrisons. In total I bought twenty-five fruit and vegetable items, both UK-grown and imported. I analysed them that same day.

Where the items were in packs, I tested two or three pieces from each. Usually the readings were similar, but two pears – purchased loose from the same supermarket box – scored 'poor' and 'excellent' (see page 20), even though they looked exactly the same. If nothing else, this aberrant result demonstrates the huge variation in nutritional quality that can occur in items of produce that look similar.

I don't claim that my survey was in any way failsafe. For a

start my selection of fruits and vegetables was purely arbitrary. They were chosen on one day in March. Perhaps the results would have been different a week later, though I somehow doubt it. What the survey showed was how far the quality of everyday foods has fallen since the wealthy nations replaced 'good husbandry' with industrial agriculture.

My results were grouped under four quality headings – poor, average, good and excellent, as suggested by Carey Reams, who used the Brix refractometer to test the quality of fruit juices in the 1960s. Based in Orlando, Florida, Reams worked chiefly with citrus growers, though he provided a consultancy service for farmers growing a wide range of crops.

The Reams's chart (shown on facing page) ranks fresh foods according to the refractive indices of their juices. Had Weston Price taken a refractometer with him on his visits to remote and healthy communities, the chances are their foods would have fallen into the 'excellent' category.

Foods scoring 'excellent' are most likely to be rich in minerals and antioxidants. They are also the foods that taste good. Of almost a hundred pieces of fruit and vegetable tested in my Somerset survey, only one – a pear – came out as 'excellent'. No less than 70 per cent of the foods tested fell into the 'poor' or 'average' categories. These are foods too low in nutrients to promote good, long-term health.

Undoubtedly the best foods – those scoring 'excellent' on the Reams chart – are the ones most likely to deliver both sound nutrition and a good flavour. As I discovered, those rated as 'good' can also be tasty, and probably supply an acceptable level of nutrition. But foods rated as 'average' or 'poor' are hardly worth eating.

According to my small-scale survey, more than two-thirds of the fresh produce sold in our local supermarkets on that March day was sub-standard. Though the big retailers make a show of their support for government 'healthy eating' campaigns, the foods they supply are often deficient in the very qualities that make them special. And what's equally bad, these degraded foods taste bad.

Reams's Chart: The Refractive Index of Crop Juice – Calibrated in degrees Brix

	Poor	Average	Good	Excellent		Poor	Average	Good	Excellent
FRUIT					**VEG.**				
Apples	6	10	14	18	Asparagus	2	4	6	8
Avocados	4	6	8	10	Beets	6	8	10	12
Bananas	8	10	12	14	Bell peppers	4	6	8	12
Cantaloupe melons	8	12	14	16	Broccoli	6	8	10	12
Casaba melons	8	10	12	14	Cabbage	6	8	10	12
Cherries	6	8	14	16	Carrots	4	6	12	18
Coconut	8	10	12	14	Cauliflower	4	6	8	10
Grapes	8	12	16	20	Celery	4	6	10	12
Grapefruit	6	10	14	18	Corn stalks	4	8	14	20
Honeydew melons	8	10	12	14	Corn (young)	6	10	18	24
Kumquats	4	6	8	10	Cow peas	4	6	10	12
Lemons	4	6	8	12	Endives	4	6	8	10
Limes	4	6	10	12	English peas	8	10	12	14
Mangoes	4	6	10	14	Field peas	4	6	10	12
Oranges	6	10	16	20	Green beans	4	6	8	10
Papayas	6	10	18	22	Hot peppers	4	6	8	10
Peaches	6	10	14	18	Kohlrabi	6	8	10	12
Pears	6	10	12	14	Lettuce	4	6	8	10
Pineapples	12	14	20	22	Onions	4	6	8	10
Raisins	60	70	75	80	Parsley	4	6	8	10
Raspberries	6	8	12	14	Peanuts	4	6	8	10
Strawberries	6	10	14	16	Potatoes	3	5	7	8
Tomatoes	4	6	8	12	Potatoes, sweet	6	8	10	14
Watermelons	8	12	14	16					
Turnip	4	6	10	12					
GRASSES					Squash	6	8	10	12
Alfalfa	4	8	16	22	Sweet corn	6	10	18	24
Grains	6	10	14	18	Turnips	4	6	8	10
Sorghum	6	10	22	30					

As I carried out my quality survey, I sampled every item tested. Though opinions on flavour are necessarily subjective, to me there was no question. Foods that produced a low Brix reading tasted dire.

Take the pack of Moroccan strawberries, for example. They were on sale at a reduced price in Tesco. On the Reams scale they ranked as 'poor'. They tasted watery and bland. Eating them was an unpleasant experience. By contrast, a tray of American-grown Pink Lady apples – on sale in the same store – tasted sweet and delicious. The refractometer reading put them in the 'good' category.

My survey also confirmed that the term 'organic' provides no guarantee of nutritious food. A tray of organically-grown Spanish strawberries from Sainsbury's came out as 'poor' on the Brix chart, the same category as Tesco's conventionally-grown crop.

A bag of Israeli organic oranges from Tesco were ranked as only 'average', as were the store's organically-grown carrots from Scotland. A box of organic tomatoes – grown in Spain – were classed as 'poor'. A pack of conventionally-grown carrots from Morrisons fell into the 'average' category, while UK-grown organic carrots from the same store were ranked as 'poor'.

Organic crops are produced without pesticide sprays or chemical fertilizers. But this doesn't mean the soils they're grown in will contain the right balance of minerals and trace elements to grow a healthy crop.

It used to be assumed by scientists that soil provided all the elements plants needed to grow sturdy and strong. The crop simply took up those minerals it needed. This is now known to be untrue. Some agricultural soils have long-term, structural imbalances in trace elements. Sandy or peaty soils, for example, may be deficient in copper. Manganese and boron deficiencies often occur in soils that contain large amounts of chalk or limestone.

Many more soils have had their normal mineral balance destroyed by decades of chemical farming. A change to organic methods doesn't automatically make them capable of growing healthy, well-mineralized crops.

A good supply of minerals is vital for the health of human beings – as it is for all living organisms. Life on Earth developed in the Pre-Cambrian Sea, a rich primeval soup containing the full complement of ninety or so minerals. All were incorporated in the single-cell organisms from which plants and animals evolved.

Primeval soils were so rich in minerals that trees were capable of growing up to ten metres in a single year. In the late Jurassic period, the mighty thunder lizard – *Apatosaurus* – was the size of a tennis court and weighed twenty-five tons. Yet it consumed its vegetarian diet through a mouth no bigger than that of a horse. Nutritionists estimate that to sustain such a vast animal, the plant life of the period must have contained thirty times the mineral levels of today's vegetation.

For good health, human beings need seven minerals in relatively large amounts. These are calcium, magnesium, phosphorus, potassium, sodium, sulphur and chloride,[4] the so-called macro-minerals.

In addition, the body needs a number of essential trace elements. Though they are required in only minute amounts, they are vital to the normal functioning of key metabolic processes. Essential trace elements include boron, cobalt, copper, chromium, germanium, selenium, iodine, zinc, molybdenum, silicon, manganese, iron and vanadium. The number known to be essential to life now exceeds thirty, though the exact role of many of them are not fully understood. (See table of essential minerals in Appendix I.)

A fertile soil can provide the plant with all of these. But to do so it needs to be well mineralized. It also needs a healthy structure with plenty of biological activity. Plants cannot efficiently extract trace elements from the tiny rock fragments that make up the mineral fraction of soils, though acids secreted by their roots can help to make them available.

Plants rely heavily on microscopic bacteria and fungi to release essential minerals from rock particles. Having been incorporated into microbial protoplasm, these trace elements are then circulated within the subterranean food chain until released in a form the plant can use. Without a large population of microbes, soils are physically unable to supply the plant with nutrients, even when chemical analysis may show them to be present.

This is why a rich, fertile soil is the only sure route to good health in the population living from it. This is not a new idea. Charles Northern (see box on page 24) was aware of this in the 1930s.

As early as the 1930s, an Alabama physician called Charles Northern was speaking out against the poorly-mineralized foods that many Americans were eating.

Northern specialized in biochemistry and nutritional medicine. But he gave up general practice to study ways of improving the nutritional value of foods by restoring the mineral balance of over-worked soils. His claim was that human health depended on a good supply of minerals. So the best way to build a healthy population was first to build a healthy, fertile soil.

In 1936, Northern's views were presented as testimony to a Congressional investigation into US farm practices. He said: 'The more I studied nutritional problems and the effects of mineral deficiencies upon disease, the more plainly I saw that here lay the most direct approach to better health.

'We know that vitamins are complex chemical substances, which are indispensable to nutrition . . . Disorder and disease result from any vitamin deficiency. It is not commonly realized, however, that vitamins control the body's appropriation of minerals, and that in the absence of minerals they have no function to perform.

'Lacking vitamins, the system can make some use of minerals. But lacking minerals, vitamins are useless.'

Northern was simply echoing the words of Nobel Prize-winner Alexus Carrel, a quarter of a century earlier: 'Minerals in the soil control the metabolism in plants, animals and man. All life will either be healthy or unhealthy according to the fertility of the soil.'

Minerals are in our foods today because of events that took place more than 10,000 years ago, at the end of the last ice age. As the glaciers retreated, they exposed the fine dust produced by the grinding action of ice on the rocks below. This mineral-rich dust was spread by the wind across the surface of the planet, re-mineralizing soils and producing a burst of biological activity.

Three thousand years after glaciation, soils across the

Earth's land surface reached an average depth of almost two metres. Today the average soil depth is just 12 centimetres. In the mineral-enriched soils, trees could grow to massive proportions. In the pre-historic forest of post-glacial Europe, trees grew trunks that measured 23 metres to the first branch.[5]

The legendary 'giant elk' of Ireland – *Megaloceros giganteus* – stood two metres tall at the shoulders, the male carrying a set of antlers spanning three metres from tip to tip.[6] In reality it was no elk, but a deer. Nor was it confined to Ireland. In the late Pleistocene epoch, it ranged widely throughout northern Europe and Asia. Each year the male would shed its antlers, growing in their place an even bigger set. To support such a huge physiological demand, the vegetation eaten by the animal must have contained high concentrations of calcium and other minerals – the gift of a fertile, mineral-rich soil.[7]

Over the past 5,000 years, the glacial minerals have been steadily washed from the soil. This is a natural process of demineralization, brought about chiefly by the action of rainwater on soil. But over the past four decades, the whole process has been cranked up by the rise of chemical farming.

Traditional farming methods aimed to retain minerals in the topsoil. By returning plant and animal wastes to the land, communities were able to slow mineral loss – or even stop it altogether. Farmers would also add natural mineral fertilizers to the land. The aim was to boost levels of trace elements, or to improve soil structure so minerals could be more easily taken up by plants. One of the earliest forms of fertilizer used by British farmers was marl – a soft, clay soil rich in calcium. Later they began spreading chalk or ground limestone to the land. In the first half of the twentieth century, basic slag (see page 177) – a by-product of steel making – became a popular fertilizer. Besides calcium and phosphorus, it added a large number of trace elements to the soil (see page 23).

The era of chemical farming put an end to these traditional materials. Farmers came to rely on manufactured inorganic chemicals to stimulate the growth of their crops. Far from enhancing fertility, the new chemical fertilizers hastened the loss of trace elements from soil, or so damaged its structure that they were no longer accessible to plants.

As the mineral content of soils fell, so did their levels in everyday foods. That's why the legacy of chemical farming is a nation overwhelmed by sickness.

The country road from Pitlochry to Strathardle in Perthshire takes you through some of the most desolate and barren countryside in Scotland. Winding through Glen Brerachen, the road follows the river between the high peaks of Ben Vrackie and Creag Dhubh on the southern slopes of the Grampian Mountains.

A less promising place to grow food crops would be hard to imagine. This glen was once covered in forest. Now the land is exposed to the full might of the Scottish winter. With many of its nutrients washed away, the soil has grown acid and sour. Coarse upland grasses clothe the hillside that once grew good potato crops.

But a remarkable couple – Cameron and Moira Thomson – have made this desert bloom again. They've found a way to grow superb vegetables – large cabbages and onions, while their greenhouses and polytunnel grow crops of tomatoes, cucumbers, sweetcorn, squashes, courgettes and marrows.

The secret of the Thomsons' gardening success is simple – so simple that it's hard to grasp the importance of what they've done. There among the heathers and the tussocky grasses they have created a fertile soil. And they've proved that it's a good soil – not chemicals – that grows healthy crops.

As you walk up the farm lane from the little carpark at Ceanghline, Straloch Farm, near Enochdhu, you know you're witnessing something remarkable. Even on a rainy day the terraced gardens stand out like oases in the desert. Amid the drab green of the upland grassland, they are filled with tall, brightly-coloured flowers and healthy vegetables.

The soil they're growing in is dark and slightly gritty to the touch. The Thomsons mix it themselves before spreading it on to their garden terraces. It's made from fine rock dust hauled from a nearby quarry, and compost made from green waste by Dundee City Council. Together the two ingredients produce ideal conditions for healthy crop growth. The dust – from the volcanic rock basalt – supplies minerals that rainfall and chemical farming have stripped out of many soils. Compost provides organic matter for microbial activity, the prerequisite of a fertile soil.

With their rock dust and compost mix, the Thomsons have produced an 'instant soil' – fertility on tap. And they've done it by copying nature. They have effectively reproduced post-glacial conditions on their worn-out twenty-first-century hillside. They have shown that on a soil rich in minerals, and well endowed with organic matter, it's possible to grow large, healthy crops without the arsenal of chemical fertilizers and pesticides used by commercial farmers today.

If soil minerals can produce a harvest like that high on a Scottish hillside, they'll transform the health and yields of crops across the country, says the couple. And this in turn will lead to a healthier, happier population. Cameron says: 'For years people have dismissed us as cranks and loonies. How can it be possible to change the world simply by spreading a bit of rock dust on the ground? But it's nature's way, and it works.

'The life on this planet is sustained by the minerals in the soil. When they're gradually lost through natural leaching or intensive chemical farming, things start to go wrong. That's the reason why we're so unhealthy – why the whole food chain is unhealthy. But if we're prepared to take account of nature we can quickly get things back on track. This is the way we can be healthy again.'

Bringing fertility back to a Scottish glen has been no easy undertaking for the Thomsons. For most of their adult lives, the two former art students have struggled to find a way of living that didn't harm the planet. Back in the 1980s they lived in a small cottage on a farm near Dundee. At the time their first child was born, they were trying hard to become self-sufficient, growing all their own food organically.

Though they worked long hours in their garden with traditional organic methods, it failed to produce the quality crops they believed it should. Plants were prone to pests and disease, and the soil seemed to be lacking some vital nutrient. Something was out of kilter, as if the productive power of the land were being held in check. At the same time the two had begun to notice subtle climate changes that were affecting the plants around them.

By chance they listened to a radio review of a book by two American authors, John Hamaker and Don Weaver (see Chapter 11). Titled *The Survival of Civilization*, the book proposed the re-mineralization of farms and gardens with fine rock dust as a way of combating global warming. Spreading rock dust on the land would produce an upsurge in biological activity, the writers argued. As the silicate rock weathered, carbon dioxide would be taken from the atmosphere and 'locked up' by the formation of calcium and magnesium carbonates. At the same time the release of trace elements would produce bigger and healthier crops.

To Cameron and Moira the idea came as a revelation. Here was an explanation for their faltering crops. Might it be that their land had become depleted of essential trace elements? They decided to give rock dust a try.

In the book Hamaker and Weaver had recommended finely-ground glacial gravel as the best material to use. This is the dust created when large glaciers crush the rocks beneath them. Such gravels usually represent a number of different rock types, so they're likely to produce a broad spectrum of soil minerals.

Cameron Thomson went to a number of quarries for his dust. He had no less than twenty tons of it ploughed into the quarter-acre garden. To provide the necessary organic matter he grew 'green manure' crops of radish and vetch, digging them in by hand. Once the ground had been prepared, he began growing fruit and vegetables on the freshly-'mineralized' plot.

The results were immediate. The Thomsons began harvesting unusually large cabbages and cauliflowers, gooseberries and blackcurrants that were filled with flavour. No fertilizers or chemicals were used, and the crops never needed watering, such was the moisture-holding capacity of the reinvigorated soil.

Neighbours started to take an interest in the rock dust phenomenon. Soon the garden they had named the Earth Regeneration Centre was receiving intrigued visitors. Many went home determined to re-mineralize their own gardens.

But the couple had wider ambitions. They wanted to test the system under tougher conditions, and at the same time reveal its benefits to a bigger audience. That's when they had a piece of good luck.

Among their visitors was a sympathetic landowner who offered them – rent free – seven acres below the crag face of Creag Dhub, high in the Perthshire hills, 1,000 ft feet above sea level. Here at Ceanghline they opened the Sustainable Ecological Earth Regeneration contro – the SEER Contre. And here is where mixtures of rock dust and composts have made the worn-out soils of this Scottish glen bloom again.

At Straloch Farm the Thomsons set out to test a simple but compelling idea. The results in this lonely Scottish glen look convincing. Now there's an urgent need to research the technique on a wider scale under commercial farming conditions. If it had involved a potentially-profitable chemical fertilizer instead of a relatively cheap, natural product, no doubt the research would have been completed long ago.

As mentioned earlier in this chapter (see pages 15–17), the link between human health and minerals in the soil was highlighted by the American dentist Weston A. Price in his book *Nutrition and Physical Degeneration*. He cites as an example a glacier which, during the last ice age, covered one-half of the state of Ohio. It occupied an area west of a line starting east of the city of Cleveland and extending diagonally across the state to Cincinnati.

At the time Price was writing, human degenerative conditions were higher in areas south and east of this line than in areas that had been covered by the glacier thousands of years earlier. For example, infant mortality was 50 per cent higher in the non-glacial areas than in the glaciated parts of the state.

According to Price this was the result of the poorer miner-alization of soils in non-glaciated areas.

Price also studied the American Heart Association's figures for death rates from heart disease across the United States during the 15 years leading up to the Second World War. He found that in some regions they were higher by more than 50 per cent, the rises being greatest in areas that had been under human occupation for the longest period – New England, the states bordering the Great Lakes, and the Pacific Coast states. Through demineralization these soils had gradually lost their capacity for maintaining human and animal health.

'This is one of the evils that has accompanied our progress in modernization,' wrote Price. 'We do not realize how much modern human beings are handicapped and injured since they learned how to modify nature's foods.'

3
The Illusion of Plenty

Strung out along the Ohio River valley in the eastern United States, are a series of earthworks left behind by a long-extinct tribe of native Americans. Archaeologists know them as 'the mound builders'. Among their structures is a burial site thought to have been used for more than 1,500 years. This ancient cemetery contains bones left during much of that time.

Scientists looking for disease patterns found little of interest among the earliest bone fragments. These dated from a time when the tribe were living as hunter-gatherers, subsisting mainly on buffalo meat and the roots, herbs and berries they gathered from the native prairie grassland.

But bones dating from a later period showed signs of many chronic diseases, including juvenile anaemia, arthritis, TB and osteoporosis. The physical decline began at a time when the tribe were undergoing a fundamental change in their way of life. They had given up hunting and were settling down to be farmers. This, it seems, is when their troubles began.

In modern Britain most of us think of western agriculture as a success story. Today's farmers feed twice as many people as they did before the Second World War. With sophisticated machinery and the latest farm chemicals they produce vast amounts of food with an ever-dwindling labour force. Never in the nation's history has so much wheat poured into the grain silos; never have so many bulk milk tankers lumbered up and down the motorways delivering 'the white stuff' to processing dairies.

Yet amid all this plenty, British people are suffering much sickness. The conditions that afflict us today are not the great infectious diseases of old – cholera, typhoid, diphtheria and TB. Instead we're succumbing to what the health authorities term 'the diseases of civilization': diseases that result not from invasion by pathogenic organisms but from a collapse in the body's own support systems.

The names of today's illnesses are frighteningly familiar – coronary heart disease, cancer, diabetes, arthritis, osteoporosis, Alzheimer's and depression. Hardly anyone in western society remains untouched by them. In Britain – as in the United States – one in three of us will develop cancer. Half the population are likely to suffer from heart disease during their lifetime, and one-third of the population will develop an allergy.

Learning disabilities such as dyslexia and hyperactivity now blight the lives of tens of thousands of youngsters. At the other end of life, nine out of ten people will suffer the pain of arthritis by the time they reach sixty.

Despite this grim litany, health statistics show we are continuing to live longer. What the figures don't reveal is the massive increase in intervention medicine it takes to keep us going. Multiple bypass surgery, chemotherapy and an avalanche of therapeutic drugs are prolonging our lives. But they don't protect us from years of pain and disability.

In his book *Health Defence*, medical pharmacologist Paul Clayton describes the majority of seemingly healthy adults as 'the pre-ill'.

Their bodies contain the seeds of diseases that will eventually lay them low and may even kill them. Unseen, an artery is starting to silt up; bones are thinning; brain cells are dying. In time they will lead to heart attack, bone fractures and dementia.

Human beings are programmed for long, healthy and active lives. The oldest person ever recorded – the French woman Jeanne Calment, from Arles – died in 1997 at the age of 122.[1] Far from being a health fanatic, she had drunk two glasses of port daily for most of her life, and had given up smoking only five years before her death. Her diet is largely unrecorded, but it's likely to have included a substantial number of healthy foods. Sadly many foods that were once considered 'healthy' have undergone a subtle but damaging change.

It would be hard to imagine a healthier environment than the small Perthshire town of Aberfeldy. With its handsome, stone-built commercial centre, it stands alongside the sparkling River Tay, amid a countryside of pastureland and oakwoods. On both sides of the valley, the hills rise steeply to the crags and moors of the southern Highlands.

It would seem the ideal place to bring up children. Here, surely, youngsters can grow up robust and happy, with the expectation of long, active lives. But clean air and crystal clear lochs are no protection against the diseases of civilization. This little town has its full share of human misery.

Until he retired in the early 1980s, Walter Yellowlees had been a doctor in the town for almost thirty years. He first qualified during the Second World War and signed up in the Army Medical Corps. As a medical officer with the Cameron Highlanders, he witnessed some of the bloodiest battles of the war. When hostilities ended, he joined the small rural practice at Aberfeldy and there he saw a different kind of tragedy.

The upper Tay Valley he found in those early post-war years still supported a scattering of small, family farms. Most were mixed farms, their tenants combining stock rearing with a traditional form of crop rotation. The whole system was aimed at maintaining – and sometimes improving – the natural fertility of the soil.

But by the time he retired, the small farms had mostly gone. So had the practice of mixed farming. The new lairds of the Tay Valley were large, specialist farmers. Their fields had become monocultures, worked by sophisticated machines and goaded into ever-higher levels of production by heavy dressings of chemical fertilizer. They were producing not for their local community but for a distant commodity market.

With the ending of local food production came a mounting toll of degenerative diseases. Coronary heart disease – virtually unknown before the 1920s – began striking down people who in other ways seemed perfectly fit. Clean air and hard physical work offered little protection. Heart disease was as likely to strike the shepherd or gamekeeper in the tranquil Highland glen, as the stressed commuter caught up in the rush and din of the city. And along with heart disease came a host of gastro-intestinal conditions, from constipation to peptic ulcers and bowel cancer.

The GP quickly formed his own view on the cause of all this misery – the steady erosion of the ancestral Scottish diet. In the mid-nineteenth century, most rural Scots enjoyed robust good health, often well into old age. Their foods were the foods of the Scottish countryside produced by a farming system still dedicated to fertile soils.

Among the staple dietary items were oatmeal, potatoes, turnips, kale, cheese, butter, milk and ale. On these locally-grown and nourishing foods country people stayed healthy, often living to great ages. Historical records for the parish of Fortingall – to the west of Aberfeldy – showed that in the final decade of the eighteenth century, many residents were old, and some very old. There were a good number of octogenarians, a handful of people in their nineties, and even a few who had topped the century.

The rot began with the coming of the railway in 1867. Trains brought in cheap processed foods – sugar, margarine, and white flour, stripped of its nutrient-rich bran. The traditional Scottish high tea metamorphosed into a feast of starch and sugar – scones, jam, cakes and biscuits. The dangers of such foods were spelled out by one of Yellowlees' great mentors, Surgeon Captain T. L. Cleave, in his book *The Saccharine Disease*.[2]

From his rural practice, Yellowlees became an outspoken critic of industrial foods. When the human body became overloaded with refined carbohydrates, he argued, conditions like diabetes, coronary disease, ulcers and colon cancer were the likely consequences.

But there was powerful opposition to the theory. Medical chiefs on both sides of the Atlantic had latched on to an opposing idea, one that linked heart disease and many cancers to saturated fats, especially animal fats.

Traditional foods like beef, butter, eggs and whole milk began to be stigmatized. The powerful margarine industry weighed in with well-funded campaigns promoting low-fat spreads in place of butter. To Yellowlees the case was bogus. Were we really to believe that traditional foods – prized over the centuries for their health-giving qualities – had suddenly become the cause of catastrophic death and disability?

In 1978 – with the argument raging – he was invited to deliver the annual James MacKensie Lecture to the College of General Practitioners. He called his lecture 'Ill fares the land'. In it he dismissed what he called 'the dogma of animal fat'. Instead he restated his belief that traditional foods grown on fertile soils would protect against the great disease scourges of the age.

He concluded: 'The new epidemics of degenerative disease are not inevitable, nor is their cause mysterious. They are nature's language telling eloquently of our failure to understand the supreme importance of her laws.'

His GP audience listened with less than rapt attention, more a polite scepticism. When he sat down the applause was courteous rather than appreciative. But he remained undeterred. Three decades later he holds to his view as strongly as ever. And the scepticism of his medical colleagues has at last begun to melt away. The deadly consequences of industrial food – and the industrial farming that produces it – are apparent for all to see in the over-flowing surgeries and hospital clinics.

Yellowlees saw the disaster unfolding in his daily dealings with patients amid the Perthshire hills and glens. He later wrote about them in his book, *A Doctor in the Wilderness*. It is the story of a tragedy. For all the hardships of their everyday lives, the people of this Highland community had once flourished on the produce of their own fields. Then came the foods

of an urban industrial culture, and within a couple of generations the robust health of the community had begun to decline.

In his James MacKensie lecture, Yellowlees reported on the
cancer incidence in his own small rural practice of 3,500
people. Over a three-year period there had been fifty-one
new cases, many of which were of bowel cancer.[3] He also
looked at the ailments that kept working males off work. The
most common cause was bronchitis, followed by diseases of
the circulatory system – heart disease and angina. The third
most common causes of sick leave were arthritis and rheuma-
tism.

At a time of unparalleled living standards and technological
advance in medicine, Yellowlees believed he was witnessing
human decay on a massive scale – decay of teeth, arteries,
bowels and joints.

Today the upper Tay Valley remains a tranquil and beautiful
place. Dr Yellowlees took me on an introductory tour of the
local countryside. We drove along the main road to Ballinluig
as it snaked its way through oakwoods and past open fields
running down to the gleaming river.

We were just a few miles from the hillside where Cameron
and Moira Thomson were producing magnificent vegetables
with the aid of rock dust (see Chapter 2). No landscape in
Britain was in greater need of re-mineralization than this
peaceful countryside of the Tay Valley.

Most of the land was laid down to grass. Gone were the fields
of oats that had provided generations of Scots with nourishment.
Gone, too, were the fresh vegetables that had helped to make
cancer and heart disease rare conditions. Nor was there any sign
of the famous red-and-white Ayrshire cows, whose creamy,
nutrient-rich milk once went on the breakfast porridge and
supplied a dozen farmhouse dairies making butter and cheese.

The fields were now in a monoculture of industrial grasses,
heavily dosed with chemical fertilizers. Rather than produce
food for the local community, the farms of the Tay Valley are
now in the business of producing cheap raw materials for the
food manufacturing industry. The concentration of food retailing in the hands of a few major multiples – with their

centralized distribution points – has also created a demand for bulk, year-round supplies of uniform produce.

As we drove around the quiet Perthshire countryside, we talked about an earlier medical pioneer who had explored the links between food and health (see box).

Robert McCarrison – a doctor in the Indian medical service during the early 1900s – made his name for research into diseases caused by nutrient deficiencies. For a time he served in the Northwest Frontier region. There he was struck by the robust health and vitality of local communities, particularly a hill people called the Hunzas, who lived in the Karakoram Range of the Himalayas, between Pakistan, Afghanistan, China and India. They seemed to suffer none of the afflictions of industrial nations; there was no cancer, no heart disease, no diabetes, not even tooth decay. Most remained in vibrant health throughout their long lives. By contrast, the peoples of southern India suffered high mortality rates.

Later in his career, McCarrison proved that the health of the northern Hunza people was due not to any accident of genetics but to good food. As India's director of nutrition research, he set up an experiment in which a colony of rats were fed on foods typical of the northern hill people's diet. A second group were given foods like those of the south.

The Hunzas were expert farmers. They needed to be. Land was scarce in this hilly region of India. Their food was mostly grown on high, terraced gardens. All waste materials were carefully composted and returned to the land. As a result, their soils remained fertile and healthy even though they were expected to produce large amounts of food.

Most carbohydrates in the Hunza diet were in the form of whole-grain cereals. People ate no sugar or refined flour. Their protein came mainly from milk and dairy products such as butter and cheese. They ate a little meat – about one meal a week. This basic ration was supplemented with a variety of fruit and vegetables, many of which were eaten raw.

There was another, hidden benefit of their foods. The Hunza people irrigated their highland terraced gardens with the cream-coloured water from glacial streams. It was a rich source of minerals, released from the volcanic dust that had been held for millennia in the ice.

Here was a major reason for the legendary health and stamina of the Hunzas. Like the remote communities visited by the dentist Weston A. Price in the 1930s, their foods were enriched with high levels of essential trace elements.

This was the diet McCarrison fed to one little colony of laboratory rats. On it they remained vigorous and active from one generation to the next. But the group fed on a diet typical of poor people in the south of the country – in which polished rice was the main ingredient – failed to thrive. Their physique was poor and they quickly developed respiratory infections and intestinal conditions. Similar ailments appeared in rats fed on diets typical of poor people in Britain at the time – white bread, margarine, jam, tinned meat, boiled potatoes and sweet tea.

In 1936, McCarrison published his findings in his Cantor Lectures before the Royal Society of Arts. They were later published in his book, *Nutrition and Health*.[4] He expected an excited response from the medical profession, but the findings were largely ignored. Physicians were too preoccupied with disease and its treatment to pay much attention to this clue to prevention. A revolutionary group of drugs called the sulphonamides had burst on to the scene.[5] The way ahead seemed to lie with new, miracle drugs and innovative surgical techniques. The health benefits of good food seemed dull by comparison.

Within a few years, the post-war Labour government began planning its most ambitious project – a free health service for the nation. The health reformers might easily have taken McCarrison's advice and made sound nutrition and disease prevention the basis of the new service. Instead they designed it around the treatment of illness.

Following the discovery of penicillin during the war, a stream of new compounds flowed from the pharmaceutical industry. The antimicrobial streptomycin promised an end to the scourge of TB, particularly when used along with para-amino salicylic acid (PAS), a compound closely related to aspirin. It was quickly followed by tranquillizers, anti-coagulants, the anti-inflammatory hormone cortisone, and drugs to reduce high blood pressure. There seemed little that the new wonder compounds couldn't achieve.

In *The Rise and Fall of Modern Medicine*, James Le Fanu observes that the therapeutic revolution of the post-war years was not ignited by a major scientific insight.[6] Through the discovery of the sulphonamides, penicillin and cortisone, doctors and scientists had come to realize they didn't need any deep understanding of the diseases they were attempting to combat. Synthetic chemistry – blindly and randomly – would deliver the remedies that had eluded them for centuries. It was a period of supreme optimism.

In the Scottish Highlands, Yellowlees wrote that both doctors and patients had become 'dazzled by these bright, gleaming swords'. They were unaware of one simple fact – that many crippling diseases need never have been the scourges they later became. Decent housing and good nutrition could have held them in check.

It's one of the ironies of post-war Britain, that even as the policy-makers were planning their bold new health service, another branch of Whitehall was preparing to debase the nation's food. It was the 1947 Agriculture Act that drove farmers down the road of chemical production and turned them from growers of food into producers of raw materials for the food manufacturing industry.

More than half a century later, the disease statistics still head obdurately upwards. Between 1971 and the early 1990s, the numbers of newly-diagnosed cancer cases went up by 45 per cent for men and by 55 per cent for women.[7] While deaths from coronary heart disease have begun falling, it continues to afflict a growing number of people. Today, the disease accounts for one-third of premature deaths in men and one-quarter of premature deaths in women.[8] At the same time, more than two million people in the UK face life with coronary heart disease.

Over the thirteen years to 2004, the UK incidence of diabetes rose by 65 per cent for men and 25 per cent for women. The number of people with the condition – which frequently leads to heart disease – is expected to reach three million by 2010. Osteoporosis is now the cause of bone fractures in one-third of women over fifty, and one-fifth of men.[9]

In the meantime, health spending soars. In 1973, UK spending on the NHS and private health totalled £3.2 billion, equal to 4.4 per cent of the country's gross domestic product.[10] By 2004, health spending had risen to £98 billion, accounting for 8.5 per cent of GDP.

There's talk of magic bullets and revolutionary gene therapies in an echo of the 1940s when medical researchers heralded the new miracle cures that lay 'just around the corner'. Meanwhile, soils collapse under the relentless assault of chemical fertilizers and pesticides, removing any possibility of healthy food.

It's sometimes hard to comprehend the pace and scale of the revolution that has overtaken the countryside. Anyone born before 1960 will have been raised largely on natural foods, grown by traditional methods. Most people born after that time will have grown up on fake food. For almost fifty years, the people of Britain – like those in other industrial countries – have been the unwitting subjects of a mass experiment on diet.

The world my brother and I were born into at the tail end of the war was still largely 'organic'. At that time the word had no meaning. This was the way all foods had been produced, from pre-history onward.

No doubt we ate our share of industrial foods – white flour, sugar and margarine – at least as far as post-war rationing would allow. But the industrial mind hadn't yet begun to debase traditional foods – the foods that were our inheritance from generations past.

Our milk was local. Three pints arrived daily on our front doorstep, the thick topping of yellow cream stretching a quarter of the way down the bottle. And this was the ordinary 'silver top' milk, not the extra-rich 'gold top' produced by Guernsey and Jersey cows.

The dairy that supplied Hawthorn Gardens in Reading – along with half the town – had been set up by a local farmer during the depression of the 1920s. The thick band of yellow cream was a good indication that our milk had come from cows grazing naturally on fertile pastureland.

Our butter – from the Co-op grocers at the end of the road – was a deep yellow colour, showing that it, too, had come from cows eating little but fresh grass. The chances are it was richly-endowed with fat-soluble vitamins and essential fatty acids.

Most of our meat was from the Co-op butcher. It's true the beef – which we ate most Sundays – probably came from South America. But the chances are it was reared on the great pampas grasslands of Argentina. Like the famous roast beef of old England, it was invariably pasture-fed, so it would have been healthy meat.

Our bread came from a bakery just five streets away, though the wheat in it is likely to have crossed the Atlantic from Canada or the United States. Even so, it was grown largely without pesticides or chemical fertilizers. Despite the 'dust bowls' of the 1930s, most mid-western farmers were still benefiting from the natural fertility of the Plains soil, built up over thousands of years by prairie grassland.

Almost everything else we ate travelled no distance at all. My grandfather, Tom, grew it in the back garden. There was a small flock of hens to supply us with eggs, and the occasional old layer for chicken stew. Alongside the chicken run, a dozen assorted fruit bushes gave us seasonal crops of raspberries, loganberries, blackcurrants and gooseberries. And a generous plot of cultivated ground provided practically all our vegetables.

It was in that little garden that I learned 'the law of return', the guiding principle observed by farmers and growers down the ages. Every so often my grandfather would spread the ground with 'muck' – chicken manure from the run; crumbly compost from the bin behind the tool-shed; or farmyard manure scrounged from heaven knows where.

Tom had himself grown up on a farm – his father was a north Berkshire farm labourer. Returning to the land any vegetable or animal waste he could get his hands on seemed as natural and inevitable as autumn rain. It was simply the way to keep soil fertile, so making sure of a healthy crop.

In return for these gifts, the ground would pay us back handsomely. Most days there'd be something to take back to the kitchen – a milky white cauliflower; a bunch of carrots, their feathery tops still attached; or a bowl of bright red tomatoes.

In this way the garden helped to feed us – my brother and me, my mum, my grandparents, Dad when he was home, and Uncle Alan.

No one thought it extraordinary that the garden should feed us, nor that its produce should keep us healthy. It was taken as read that as long as the soil was treated properly, a steady supply of wholesome fruit and vegetables was no more than we were due. My granddad had met his proper obligations to the land. So why shouldn't it feed us in return?

Today, food is different. On a sunny July morning I join the shoppers pushing their trolleys through the entrance of our local supermarket. It's not a large branch. During the winter months it's quite big enough to serve the small Somerset seaside town and its Exmoor hinterland. But in summer – when the local population is swelled by thousands of holiday-makers – the place can get pretty frenzied.

The shoppers who file in through the automatic doors expect the foods they buy to keep them healthy, but they're likely to be let down.

The yellow butter has gone. The brands in this store – including the premium brands – are a pale cream colour. The vivid yellow – characteristic of cows grazing fresh grass – is nowhere to be found. Most modern butter is made from cows kept in sheds for much of the year and fed unsuitable feeds like cereal grains and soya meal.

Today's overworked Holstein cows have been bred to produce double the yield of cows fifty years ago. Milk

produced this way can't match the health-protecting properties of milk from cows grazing fresh, species-rich pasture,
their natural food. Nor can the butter and cheese that are
made from it.

The degradation of beef has been equally relentless. In the
brightly-lit chiller cabinets, today's prime beef looks attractive
enough. But like dairy cows, beef animals are increasingly kept
in sheds or compounds, and fed on high-energy cereal rations
supplemented with soya.

Ruminant animals are meant to eat fibrous foods, not
grains. Cereals and soya produce excess acid in the rumen
(the first stomach), and put a toxic load on the liver. The meat
from cattle raised this way is loaded with saturated fats,
making it unhealthy. Compared with grass-fed beef, the poly-
unsaturates – which constitute about 10 per cent of the fats in
beef – contain too high a proportion of omega-6 fatty acids,
which have been linked to a range of inflammatory diseases,
including asthma and rheumatoid arthritis.[11]

The whole-grain products on the shelves are equally spurious. Whole grains, such as wheat, barley and oats, are an
important part of the human diet. And in my local supermarket there seem to be enough of them on offer – wholewheat bread and pasta, and whole-grain breakfast cereals.
What the packaging doesn't tell you is the grain is likely to be
depleted in minerals and carrying the residues of pesticides
applied to the growing crop as well as to the stored grain in the
silo.

Some grains come from soils so damaged by chemicals and
fertilizers that their nutrient content is dramatically reduced.
The factory processing, with heat and pressure to produce
novelty shapes, impoverishes them still further. That's why
manufacturers routinely add a few minerals and vitamins to
the finished product. It's the only way these degraded foods
can be made to seem healthy.

But the greatest deception is in the fresh produce area.
Supermarkets like to make a big show out of fresh produce.
It makes them appear caring and responsible. The moment you
push your trolley through the automatic doors, you're con-

fronted by a colourful display of vegetables, leafy salads and plump, unblemished fruits.

Despite the aura of freshness created with such care by the store managers, most of the fruits and vegetables on offer weren't grown in healthy, fertile soils.

These days no one worries too much about fertile soils. For 10,000 years, the idea of fertility preoccupied the tillers of the earth and herders of cattle over natural grasslands. They knew their very survival depended on it. And the only way to ensure it, was to obey the law of return – to carefully put back all organic wastes and so maintain the life of the soil.

Now there's a chemical substitute. Fertility comes in bags of inorganic compounds. Though it has a cost, it comes without limit. And it has changed the nature of almost every food we eat.

The first farm I worked on – like most lowland farms of the time – was a 'mixed farm'. This meant that cash crops like wheat and barley were included in the same rotation as grass leys (short-term pastures) for grazing. It was a system of farming that had been successful in Britain for two hundred years.

When a ley was ploughed up after three years or so, the land was sown with a cereal crop. With a bit of luck, this would thrive on the nutrients released into the soil through the breakdown of grass roots and manure. After two or three years in cereals, the land would be sown with grass again. And so the cycle would begin all over again.

Today, traditional mixed farming has all but disappeared. Cattle and sheep have vanished from broad swathes of the lowland landscape, to be replaced by crop sprayers. Farmers have discovered they no longer need manure – or the broken-down roots of pasture plants – to grow heavy crops of cereals.

For the first time in human history, they can practise 'stock-less farming', confident that there'll be something to harvest. And the reason they can go on taking a crop year after year is because of the invention of a German chemist almost a century ago.

When I started working on the farm, the first job I was ever given was muck spreading. These days the very words sound like a gag from a stand-up in the Comedy Store.

My job was to haul manure that had been steaming gently all summer in a heap in the yard, and to spread it on a ley that was due to be ploughed up and sown with wheat. Time after time I would back up my tractor with its battered side-delivery muck-spreader. Then, using the small yard tractor with its front-end loader I'd fill it with steaming waste, piling it high until the lid would barely close.

Out in the field, I'd slip the tractor into low gear and engage the power take off. As I moved across the turf the rotor shaft would rumble and groan beneath three tons of well-rotted farmyard manure. Then with a roar the chains would break free, filling the air with a blizzard of brown clods.

For ten solid days I did that job. And on the bus going home each night no one wanted to sit near me.

In those far-off days, muck spreading remained one of the most important jobs on the farming calendar. Farmers knew – as my granddad had done – that the land needed its helping of organic matter if it was to stay healthy and productive. Organic matter provided the vital 'feedstock' for the billions of soil micro-organisms that play a key role in the cycling of essential minerals, making them available for growing crops.

Drive around the countryside in spring and you'll see, stacked up in almost every farmyard you pass, squat 'dumpy' bags of the kind that builders' merchants deliver small amounts of gravel in.

The bags contain chemical fertilizers, often in the form of small white pellets the size of hailstones. These contain the chemical salts of one or more of the three main plant nutrients – nitrogen, phosphorus and potassium. Of the three, nitrogen is the most important.

Nitrogen fertilizers are made by superheating two gases, nitrogen and hydrogen, in a high-pressure combustion chamber. The process – developed shortly before the First World War – won the Nobel prize for its inventor, the brilliant German chemist, Fritz Haber (see page 156). More than anything, it was this development that set British agriculture on its path to destruction.

The 1960s were a decade that gets a lot of people worked up. Some say it was a time of personal liberation, others that it was a period of unparalleled selfishness, greed and falling standards. But the sexual revolution wasn't the only social upheaval of the 1960s. This was also the decade when food went chemical.

Look in any children's book about a farm and it's likely to be portrayed in the traditional way. There'll be cows, sheep and pigs, together with a few hens scratching about in the yard and perhaps a couple of ducks on the pond. On the same farm, there'll be fields of wheat rippling in a summer breeze in a landscape of neat hedgerows.

As a picture of modern farming it's about as accurate as Constable's cornfield. Today, cattle and sheep have gone from wide stretches of the British countryside. So have the hedges that were once needed to keep them in.

Thanks to the little white prills of nitrogen fertilizer, farmers no longer need livestock manure to grow a large crop. Year after year they can fill their giant grain silos, using little more than a few bags of commercial fertilizer and the pesticide sprayer. For a quarter of a century, their main worry has been how to dispose of surplus yields without sending the price tumbling.

Long before Fritz Haber developed his historic process, farmers knew that nitrogen compounds could induce a sudden flush of plant growth. In the nineteenth century many used sodium nitrate from Chile or ammonium salts recovered from gasworks or coking ovens (see box).

Most modern farmers routinely manage their crops using chemical fertilizers. Every year they spread the little white granules, particularly nitrogen in the form of ammonium

A nineteenth-century pioneer of chemical agriculture wrote to a farming journal after treating his sheep pasture. He admitted he'd been unaware 'that agricultural products raised with heavy dressings of nitrogenous manure are always of inferior quality and unwholesome for livestock'. He continued, 'If ammonia, which is extremely soluble, be presented in excess when compared with the other elements of their growth, the result is that sap is circulated through the plant of too stimulating character. This produces in the vegetable organisms results similar to those too often observed in the human subject who imbibes too much soluble matter of a stimulating kind   high colour and vigorous vitality, but with a tendency to premature decay. In short, plants so treated are on the high road to gout.'

nitrate or urea. They produce a flush of leafy growth. But it's an unhealthy form of growth with an imbalance of minerals and cell walls that are unusually thin.

The plant is weakened and prone to disease. That's why farmers are forever spraying their crops with fungicides. It's good business for the chemical industry. But as a way of growing healthy food it's seriously flawed.

Chemical fertilizers have created the illusion of plenty. But that's all it is, an illusion. For the grains that fill the silos – like the fruit and vegetables on the supermarket shelves – are not real foods. They are subtly but significantly different from what went before.

4
The Nutrients We Need

It is the very heart of pastoral England – a gently rolling ocean swell of hedges, spinneys and green fields. The neat, ordered landscape seems the quintessence of fullness and plenty.

It's true there are rather more arable crops than there used to be – and fewer pasture fields. A century ago this would have been a countryside of mixed farming. Still it would be hard to think of a more promising place to grow food than this corner of east Leicestershire in the nation's heartland. But, for livestock, this countryside holds a sinister threat (see box).

Farm animals are among the victims of industrial agriculture. Many of them suffer sickness and disease from eating grass and forage crops depleted of nutrients. Most farm livestock are slaughtered young, before any symptoms begin to show. But if they were allowed to live out their natural lives, there's little doubt they'd suffer from the same crippling disease epidemic as the human population.

After all, animals and humans alike live on crops from the same over-exploited soils. The land that robs wheat and other crops of nutrients is also feeding livestock. Some day the wheat will be on sale in cafes and supermarkets as bread or breakfast cereals, or maybe a tempting gateau. And even before the food processors got hold of it, it'll have been robbed of many of its health-giving nutrients.

Close to the village of Tilton-on-the-Hill in Leicestershire, Ian Farnsworth rears prime lamb on his lush green pastureland, just a few miles from the busy A47 trunk road. It's a job he takes seriously. His strong, well-fleshed Charollais-cross lambs are as good as any you'll see in the county. But to get them that way he first had to track down a mystery ailment that blighted his farm and all it produced.

For some time he had been aware that things weren't quite as they should be at Manor Farm. Throughout the spring and summer he was putting sizeable doses of nitrate fertilizer on to his grassland. Yet despite the resulting flush of grass, his lambs failed to thrive.

While most of the single lambs would fatten up well enough, twin lambs needed a lot of extra 'concentrate' feeds (high-energy cereals) to make the grade. At the same time, too many of his ewes and their offspring seemed to be hobbling around with foot ailments.

Others displayed a yellowing of the wool, a condition that seemed linked to an unusual flakiness of the skin. Ian put it down to dermatitis. But he wasn't happy about it. In a host of small ways his animals seemed unhealthy and out-of-sorts.

By chance he heard about a talk being organized by a local farmers' discussion group. It was on the subject of soil minerals, the essential trace elements so vital for the growth and health of both plants and animals. As a result of what he heard he had his soils tested. They were found to be deficient in a number of elements, including selenium, copper, zinc and iodine.

It was a discovery that was to transform the fortunes of the farm – and the quality of the meat sold from it. He quickly arranged for his fields to be spread with a mineral supplement to make good the deficiencies in the soil. Almost at once the health of his animals improved dramatically.

The yellowing of the wool disappeared, and lameness and foot ailments became a rarity. The following year his ewe flock produced and reared 15 per cent more lambs than before. And all the lambs – twins included – fattened quickly on the reinvigorated pastures, without any extra 'concentrate' feeds.

Ian now uses just a quarter of the nitrate fertilizer he used to put on before discovering the 'sickness' in his soil. Even so, his pastures are more productive than ever, providing good grazing for the sheep three weeks earlier in spring and continuing to grow a month longer in the autumn.

With the soil trace elements now in balance, the amount of clover in the pasture has increased year by year. Through the action of bacteria in their roots, clover plants are able to build up nitrate levels in the soil naturally without the need for chemical fertilizer. Soon it should be possible to stop buying the bags of chemicals altogether.

'I can tell at a glance the sheep are doing far better on pasture,' says Ian. 'They have a contented look about them – a look they never seemed to have before. These days they're healthy and thriving. So the meat they produce has got to be healthier for the consumer.

'The abattoir people are happy, too. They can't seem to get enough of our lambs. So they're obviously popular with the customers. From the few we keep back for the freezer at home, I can tell you there's no sweeter-tasting lamb anywhere.'

As mentioned earlier, traditional farming systems invariably include careful provision for keeping up the level of soil minerals. Western industrial agriculture, by contrast, impoverishes its soils with a constant bombardment from chemical fertilizers and agrochemicals.

As a result, levels of organic matter in the soil have fallen relentlessly. The vital army of soil organisms are denied the essentials of life. The health and vitality of the soil begins to falter, and farmers are made more than ever dependent on the chemical companies.

At the same time, as soil doctors such as Robert Plumb will advise (see Chapter 1), fertilizers displace soil calcium, an element that plays a key role in maintaining the mineral balance and structure of soils. The healthy crumb structure breaks down, the vital air channels fill. The soil becomes compacted and sour. Sometimes alcohol and formaldehyde start to build up. Both are deadly to the normal life of a fertile soil.

At this point the farmer starts to lose money. Even the flush of chemically-induced growth starts to tail off. But the highest price is paid by the animals that eat the crops from these sick soils. And of course, by us.

A farmer friend, near where I live in Somerset, had a sudden outbreak of salmonella poisoning in his calves. He called in the vet, who prescribed antibiotics. Although half the infected calves recovered, the rest died. The disease continued to spread to healthy animals. His sheep started to be affected, too.

In desperation he called in a firm to test his land for minerals. They took soil samples, analysed them and came back with an answer – much of his land was low in the essential trace elements selenium, iodine, copper and cobalt. The firm went on to treat the soil with the missing micro-nutrients. Very quickly the health of the cattle improved. Soon the fertility of the herd was better than it had been for years. The sheep were healthier, too, with the young lambs full of vigour and eager to suckle. As if that weren't enough, my farmer friend grew a crop of winter kale that was taller than he'd ever seen. For the first time in years he didn't need to spray it with fungicide to keep it free of disease.

Only a handful of farmers have taken such a step. Many put up with unnecessarily high levels of affliction in their animals, anything from stillbirths and abortion to pneumonia. In most cases the cause is an impaired immune system brought about by low levels of one or more essential nutrients. There's no reason to believe that the impoverished soils that make animals sick aren't having a similar effect on human beings.

In 1940, the Medical Research Council published the results of a survey into the nutrient content of many everyday foods. The authors were a doctor, R. A. McCance, and a nutritionist, E. M. Widdowson. Their studies were continued over the next 51 years and were eventually taken over by the Ministry of Agriculture. During this period, a total of five reports were published of the McCance and Widdowson results.

Known as *The Composition of Foods*, the dusty reports show how mineral levels in many everyday items have fallen during a period of intensive chemical farming. This finding was made in 2003 by David Thomas, a geologist who later trained as a nutritionist. He discovered that between 1940 and 1991 vegetables had lost – on average – 24 per cent of their magnesium, 46 per cent of their calcium, 27 per cent of their iron and no less than 76 per cent of their copper.[1]

The results for two main dietary staples were even worse. Carrots lost 75 per cent of their magnesium, 48 per cent of their calcium, 46 per cent of their iron and 75 per cent of their copper. The traditional 'spud' lost 30 per cent of its magnesium, 35 per cent of its calcium, 45 per cent of its iron and 47 per cent of its copper.

According to Thomas, you'd have needed to eat ten tomatoes in 1991 to get the amount of copper a single tomato would have supplied in 1940.

The results for other produce were scarcely more comforting. Among seventeen varieties of fruit, the amounts of both magnesium and calcium were 16 per cent lower in 1991 than they had been in 1940. The zinc content was down by 27 per cent, the iron content by 24 per cent and the copper content by 20 per cent.

Even meat showed a fall in mineral levels. In a range of ten popular cuts, the iron content fell by 54 per cent and the copper content by 24 per cent.

During the period of these changes, other aspects of the British diet have undergone a seismic shift. Chapters 1 to 3 have commented on the dramatic switch to processed and fast foods, and how the raw materials they're made from are often contaminated with weedkillers, pesticides, antibiotics and hormones. The McCance and Widdowson figures prove that many are depleted of the essential minerals that are the foundation of a healthy diet.

David Thomas finds the results alarming. He says: 'Physiologically it would be hard to over-estimate the importance of minerals and trace elements. They often act as the catalyst for other nutrients the body uses to maintain good health. It is improbable that we can function at our optimum on a physical, mental and emotional level, if the foods we have available are deficient.'

Thomas's conclusions are challenged by the Institute of Food Research at Norwich. They claim the data reveal no great decline in the mineral content of fresh foods. In any case most consumers don't depend on fruit and vegetables for the minerals they contain. According to the food scientists at Norwich their importance lies in their many other dietary components such as glucosinolates, flavonoids and vitamins.

But if Thomas is right these valuable compounds are likely to be reduced, too. Minerals play a key role in most of plant enzyme systems, so if they're lacking the plant cell will be unable to manufacture its full complement of phytonutrients.

The exact role of minerals in human nutrition is still unclear. The long neglect of nutrition by orthodox medicine has left big gaps in the scientific knowledge. There's not even any agreement about which of the ninety or so trace elements found in nature can be considered 'essential' for human health. Some nutritionists believe that every living cell – whether in microbe, plant, animal or human being – require all the minerals to operate efficiently (see table of essential minerals in Appendix I).

As mentioned earlier, what is clear is that, along with the familiar minerals like iron, calcium and potassium, the human body needs a number of less well-known elements, such as boron, cobalt and germanium. These elements are required in tiny amounts. But without them – and the vitamins, which often work in tandem with them – the body's support systems begin to break down.

Some trace elements such as magnesium, zinc, iron and

selenium are essential to the normal functioning of the human immune system. But the fresh foods we now eat contain, on average, 50 per cent less than the foods of our grandparents' time. Chemical fertilizers have stripped many of these vital nutrients from the soil or blocked their uptake by plants. More are removed from crops during processing.

The element selenium is a classic example. In Britain, average intake of selenium is just 35 micrograms a day. The recommended rate for health is 150–200 micrograms.

Selenium plays a key role in the human immune system. Low blood selenium levels have been linked to heart disease[2] and most cancers.[3] Yet virtually everyone in Britain – unless they're taking mineral supplements – is likely to have low blood selenium levels. This is because most UK soils are poor in the element, as are the soils in much of Europe, and the widespread use of high-nitrogen fertilizers has made matters worse.

GP Mark Draper, an integrative physician and consultant to the food supplement company Cytoplan, is convinced that a sizeable section of the UK population suffer from type 2 malnutrition – they are deficient in essential micro-nutrients. The major nutrients such as protein, carbohydrates and fats are present in abundance – sometimes in excess. But people no longer get the essential minerals they need to stay healthy. The elements iron, zinc and selenium are the ones most likely to be in short supply.

The problem is exacerbated by the decline in average energy intakes. People engaged in hard physical work can easily utilize 4,000 calories a day.[4] That's the kind of intake that was common in Britain fifty years ago. Today, with our largely sedentary lives, most people have calorie intakes of half that or less. That means their intake of micro-nutrients is also halved. When the foods themselves have been depleted of minerals, vitamins and phytochemicals by intensive farming or processing, many people are likely to go short.

According to Draper, common signs of micro-nutrient deficiency are recurrent infections – the sort of everyday ailments that fill doctors' waiting rooms with patients seeking prescriptions for antibiotics. But there can be far more severe consequences for health. For the unborn child, a deficiency in one or more essential trace elements can lead to developmental difficulties later in the child's life. There's an increased risk of conditions such as dyslexia, Asperger's syndrome and dyspraxia.

In adults, micro-nutrient deficiency may be the cause of chronic fatigue and reduced immunity. In the elderly it leads to the common degenerative conditions like osteoporosis, Alzheimer's, cancer and cardiovascular disease. In Britain, the world's fourth largest economy – where food is cheap and plentiful – five out of six people over sixty suffer from one or more degenerative conditions.

'In the midst of all this plenty we're seeing an epidemic of these diseases,' says Draper. 'Conditions you'd expect to see only in the elderly are occurring in younger people. And all for the want of a few minerals.'

The ideal solution would be a return to well-grown wholefoods, he believes. But where these are not available there's no alternative to a good food supplement to replace the micronutrients missing from the diet.

Draper's first experience of mineral supplements came while working as a young GP in the Turks and Caicos islands in the Caribbean. School children between seven and seventeen were given regular iron supplements after a survey had shown that many were deficient in the mineral. After six weeks, the numbers of children attending out-patient clinics with skin, scalp, ear, nose and throat infections had fallen from twenty a day to just one or two. Teachers reported that, following

In his book *Rare Earth's Forbidden Cures*, Joel D. Wallach cites examples of teenage violence, which he believes could have been averted by proper nutrition. He argues that the chief cause of violence among young males is an 'explosive' mixture of testosterone, mineral deficiencies and an excess of sugar. The remedy, he says, is a diet free of sugar and supplemented with minerals (including copper, chromium, vanadium and lithium), vitamins, amino acids, and essential fatty acids.

supplementation, children were more attentive in class and their performance – especially memory and recall – had improved.

Trace element deficiencies don't just affect physical health. They're also implicated in a range of emotional and behavioural disorders. In a celebrated study at the young offenders centre at Aylesbury in Buckinghamshire, youngsters were offered dietary supplements containing minerals, vitamins and essential fatty acids.[5] At the start of the trial more than half were found to have low intakes of zinc, while three-quarters had low intakes of magnesium and almost all of them were deficient in selenium.

During the nine months of the trial, young offenders on the dietary supplement committed a quarter fewer offences than a group given dummy pills. The greatest reduction was in the number of serious offences, which fell by 40 per cent.

Deficiencies of calcium, iron, magnesium, zinc and copper all play a part in the onset of depression. Mineral and vitamin supplements have also been found to reduce rage and mood swings in children with psychiatric disorders. Poor food from degraded soils is the likely cause of many of the behavioural problems that blight the lives of thousands of youngsters.

It's not only in western countries that people are suffering the ill effects of degraded soils. The west has exported its industrial farming methods around the world, including many developing countries. Even in countries where food intake has increased, diseases linked to mineral and vitamin deficiencies remain common or have gone up.[6]

The United Nations estimates that no fewer than two billion people worldwide are suffering from iron deficiency anaemia – a condition that undermines their physical and mental health.[7] Seven hundred million people, most of them in less-developed countries, are said to suffer from iodine deficiency, the greatest preventable cause of brain damage and mental retardation.

The health consequences of chemical farming were predicted more than twenty-five years ago, by a pioneering American physician called Maynard Murray. In his research on mineral nutrition, he became interested in the reasons for the good health of sea creatures compared with creatures that lived on the land. The animals of the oceans, he discovered, suffered few of the degenerative diseases that afflicted land animals. He attributed the better health status to the higher mineral levels of sea water.

In *Sea Energy Agriculture*, published in 1976, he wrote:

When an element is leached from the land, the resulting (mineral) imbalance causes either a blocking of the other elements present so they cannot be taken up by plants, or a substitution of some other element – for the one leached – takes place. As more and more of the topsoil elements were leached away, humans began to put back manure, decayed foliate, and dead animals for fertilizer. In the process they had returned the elements to the soil in the same proportions as they had been cropped out.

In modern times agriculture has begun the process of adding the basic elements of nitrogen, phosphorus and potassium plus lime – calcium chloride – in large amounts. This has initially caused the yield from crops to increase. However, there is growing evidence that excessive build-up of these four elements blocks the uptake of vital trace elements. In essence this means that leaching away of elements and excessive application of the four macro-elements to crop reduced soil have seriously weakened our physiological food-nutrition supply to the point where it is amazing that we are able to function at all. It is no wonder that disease constantly attacks the various land organisms – including humans – in an attempt to naturally recycle the elements so that a fresh start can be made.[8]

Murray's work is explained in Chapter 11. He was not the only scientist to highlight the importance of minerals for human health. The French biochemist André Voisin had reached similar conclusions two decades earlier.

Voisin taught at the French national veterinary school and held an honorary doctorate from the University of Bonn. But at

heart he remained a farmer. A laureate member of the Aca-
demie d'Agriculture de France, his main interest was the way
soil management affected the health of people who ate the
food.

In his book, *Soil, Grass and Cancer*, first published in 1959,
Voisin wrote:

> We should meditate on the words of Ash Wednesday:
> 'Man, remember you are dust and that you will return to
> dust.' This is not merely a religious and philosophical
> doctrine but a great scientific truth. It should be engraved
> above the entrance to every faculty of medicine in the
> world. We might then remember that our cells are made
> up of mineral elements, which are to be found in the soils
> of Normandy, Yorkshire and Australia. If these 'dusts'
> have been wrongly assembled in plant, animal or human
> cells the result will be imperfect functioning.[9]

Voisin thought it extraordinary that doctors and medical
scientists around the world scarcely gave a thought to the
foods being eaten by their patients. He tells the story of a tribe
of native Americans among whom cancer was extremely rare.
The Navajos lived on a reserve straddling the states of Arizona,
Utah, Colorado and New Mexico.

Doctors working in the local hospitals observed that cancer
rates among the 8,000 or so population were unusually low.
They suspected that some special feature of the Navajo diet
might be the cause and a team of scientists were drafted in
from several states to investigate. After months of exhaustive
study the researchers published their results. They concluded
that the Navajo diet was hardly any different from that of
other sections of the population. Low cancer rates were
probably due to some unknown genetic characteristic of
the tribe.

But when Voisin read the report he found the scientists had
ignored one vital factor. They had made no reference to the
nature of the soil, nor to Navajo cultivation methods. The tribe
held strongly to the belief that they had been formed from the

'dust' of their soil. And they were in the habit of adding a little of it to their food: they would burn cedar branches and mix the resulting ash with their maize flour. They were, in effect, adding a mineral supplement to their food. Dieticians might prescribe any number of special foods, wrote Voisin, but unless they took account of the soils the foods had been grown on their results were meaningless.

At the time Voisin's books were published – the 1950s – no one took much notice of such bizarre ideas. The medical profession was firmly in thrall to the drug companies and the medical physicists. The future lay in new miracle medicines and high-tech gadgetry. Who was this farmer to suggest that doctors go out into the fields for answers to some of the twentieth century's most intractable diseases? The idea seemed preposterous. But now, with health budgets devouring ever more of the national wealth, the logic of this clear-thinking Frenchman has begun to look more compelling.

It was Voisin who made the startling proposal that chemical disorder in the soil could lead inexorably to disorder in the human cell. He was able to show that cancer was less common in areas where the soil was calcareous – lime rich – in character. He also showed that chemical fertilizers could lead to copper deficiency, and that the breakdown of normal copper metabolism in the human body might result in cancer.

Working with farm animals he found that copper deficiency in the heavily-pregnant ewe was the cause of a nervous disease called sway-back in the lamb. Sway-back, a type of paralysis, develops after breakdown of the myelin sheath, the white insulating tissue that surrounds particular nerves. Voisin established that the degenerative process began in the foetus and was the result of copper deficiency in the soil. Simply spraying pastures with a copper solution would prevent the disease.

Voisin became convinced that studies on grazing animals were the best guide to the condition of a soil and its ability to produce healthy food for people. The key intermediary was grass. Human beings got their food from a variety of sources across the world, so it was difficult to link disease with any particular soil. But the mineral balance in grass was linked directly to the health and mineral status of the soil it grew on. It was like a 'biochemical snapshot' of the soil below. And it had a profound effect on the animal grazing on that grass.

For the French biochemist the idea was no more than a modern re-interpretation of the age-old rural wisdom that 'the animal is a product of the soil'. Any organism – whether animal or human being – was a product of the environment in which it lived, particularly the soil which manufactured its nutrients.

Voisin recalled his own surprise at seeing a group of the renowned Percheron horses in the Ukraine. In their native Perche region of France the breed was big and sturdy. But the Percherons he saw in the Ukraine were very different. They had been bred from stock imported many years earlier but had adapted to poorer grazing. Though the animals still retained the shape and character of the parent breed, they were scarcely bigger than Cossack ponies.

Viewed from modern Britain it's rather disturbing to learn that our grazing livestock have been far from healthy in recent years. The 'snapshot' offered by their diseases and ailments shows that all is not well in the soil below.

Mineral supplements can be life-savers to people whose diets are deficient in one or more essential elements – and that includes most of the population of the western industrial world. But tablets are seldom a substitute for nutrient-rich foods.

In nature, no element occurs in isolation or in association with just a few others. They are invariably part of a matrix with a host of other minerals, vitamins and fatty acids. To make use of an element, humans need a number of other nutrients that would normally occur with it in the natural world.

That's why essential elements in plant form – or in animal products – are usually far more 'available' to the human body than they would be in a tablet. To be healthy we need to put the nutrients back into our everyday foods. And that means making our soils fertile again.

I caught up with Danny Goodwin-Jones at the end of a long, bone-shaking track that wound its way down a beautiful green valley in west Wales. As I pulled up outside his handsome farmhouse he stepped from the porch to greet me, a tall ebullient figure whose energy and enthusiasm belied his 75 years.

We gazed across the valley to where a small flock of sheep nibbled at the lush pasture.

'Not mine I'm afraid,' he said, anticipating my question. 'I don't have time for that sort of thing any more.' We went into the house to talk about the things he does have time for.

As it happens he has spent a good deal of his life farming. He was born and brought up on a dairy farm near Welshpool at a time when most farms operated in ways now considered organic. After a long army career he retired at the rank of colonel and bought a small farm in west Wales. This was in the mid-1970s. He was looking forward to the challenge of a new career rearing livestock.

But the second time around, farming was not as he had remembered it. His sheep fell ill and died. His prized Welsh Black cattle failed to thrive. Vets advised him 'to feed his livestock better' without explaining exactly what that meant. Nothing he tried would make the animals flourish. By the time he had reached the desperate decision to sell up, his financial reserves were practically exhausted.

But Goodwin-Jones was not the sort of man to walk away from a defeat. He would not accept that he'd been a bad farmer, and he was determined to uncover the cause of so many ailments among his stock. Then a friend – a retired agricultural adviser – suggested that a deficiency of the mineral cobalt might have been to blame. It was an element he had never even heard of. But the chance remark sparked an intense study into the role of soil minerals in animal health. Now he runs a thriving business advising worried farmers up and down the country how to cure the sickness in their livestock.

We sat at the kitchen table and looked through sheaves of thank-you letters he had received over the years from relieved farmers. There was the Cornish sheep farmer whose flock had staggered from one health crisis to the next. Ewes had died by the dozen for years and barely one in ten lambs ever reached finishing weight. At any one time almost half the flock were suffering from lameness. Though sick with worry the farmer had to endure constant complaints from passing walkers concerned about the condition of one or other of the animals.

Soil analysis revealed an imbalance of minerals, quickly corrected by soil treatment. The effect on flock health was immediate. Ewe losses fell to a fraction of their former level. Foot-rot and lameness virtually disappeared. In the year following soil treatment, 95 per cent of lambs were sold 'fat' off the farm (i.e. ready for the butcher).

A Welsh dairy farmer wrote that mastitis cases in his herd had been cut by three-quarters following the application of minerals to his soil, while the incidence of lameness had halved. Another dairy farmer reported 'a dramatic improvement in stock of all ages' following the treatment of his land with trace elements. He expressed his 'heartfelt thanks' for the advice that had transformed the financial fortunes of his farm and probably saved the business.

Over the past two decades Britain's cattle have been hit by a series of damaging epidemics beginning with 'mad cow disease', which emerged in the 1980s. Next came foot-and-mouth disease, which spread like a brush fire through the national herd in 2001.

Goodwin-Jones is convinced that impaired immunity – the result of faulty nutrition – played a part in both these epidemics. The latest disease scourge to afflict large numbers of nation's cattle is bovine TB. Farmers blame badgers for spreading the disease to their stock; badger groups blame the reckless movement of cattle. But according to Goodwin-Jones, this disease, too, is the result of degraded soils and reduced fertility.

He sees both cattle and badgers as victims of soils depleted in selenium and other trace elements. Cattle feed on grass low in essential minerals; badgers dig for worms and grub about in the same pastures. Both end up with impaired immunity leaving them defenceless whenever they come up against the ubiquitous TB bacillus.

Supporting evidence dates as far back as the 1960s. At the University of Pennsylvania, Max Lurie, Professor of Experimental Pathology, demonstrated the role of thyroid hormones in mobilizing mammalian resistance to the TB bacillus.[10] More recently, in the UK the former dairy chemist Helen Fullerton showed that to function efficiently the thyroid depends on a number of trace elements, including selenium, copper, cobalt, zinc and iodine.[11]

According to Fullerton, many of the areas of Britain and Ireland where the eradication of bovine TB is proving so intractable have soils derived from red sandstone, granite or limestone, where trace elements are often deficient or unavailable to plants. If the trace elements removed by modern, intensive farming were restored to the soil, she argues, both cattle and badgers would acquire a natural immunity to TB.

I suggested to Goodwin-Jones that since livestock were paying the price for impoverished soils, there must be a good chance that human beings were affected, too. He had no doubts.

'Just take a look at the health statistics,' he said. 'Even with all the drugs and fancy procedures, people are becoming sick prematurely. It's what we've done to our food and our soil. Not that you'd ever get the medical profession to acknowledge it. They've got too much invested in treating illness to accept such a simple and obvious solution.'

When I left he handed me a pack of mineral and vitamin supplements. He told me he recommends them to all his friends. As I walked to the car they rattled in my pocket, a plastic box of pills to replace the nutrients that chemical farming had taken out of our food.

5
Chemical Wheat Production

Wheat is as old as civilization. In Old Testament times it was wheat that filled the granaries during periods of plenty. And today it still makes up a big part of the national diet.

Each year British people eat more than five million tons of the ancient grain in one form or another. We munch it daily in bread, in breakfast cereals, in pasta, cakes and biscuits, and in a host of snack foods.

'Packed with wholewheat goodness,' says the slogan on the cereal box. And so it could be. Grown in a fertile, well-nourished soil, wholegrain wheat is rich in B vitamins and in vitamin E. It's also well endowed with trace elements – including calcium, magnesium and iron – together with a number of disease-fighting phytonutrients and antioxidants. Well-grown wheat has more of them than many fruits and vegetables.

But the wheat we eat in our daily toast and breakfast cereals has lost its power to promote health and vitality. The growers and processors of this staple food have robbed it of nutrients and laced it with chemical contaminants.

Today's wheat is the product of nineteenth-century industrial chemistry and was developed on the American plains. Now it is traded as a global raw material for edible products that have as much in common with real food as the potato crisp.

Driving through Britain's 'big wheat country' in Eastern

England in early summer you could almost believe you were crossing the prairies. In every direction the bright green crops stretch away across the boundless plain. The short, sturdy plants are packed tightly together. If there are any wild flowers to be seen, they're likely to be growing on the roadside verges. Out on the farmland there's precious little room for them – except under some EU-funded conservation scheme. For this is a landscape dedicated to production.

For the facts about modern wheat production, there's no better place to start than the annual Cereals Event in East Anglia. Traditional agricultural shows aren't much help. With their well-scrubbed cattle and speciality foods they're a great public relations exercise for the industry. But they tell you little about the real business of farming.

The wheat farmer's programme begins in the autumn when the plants are still very small. First they're sprayed with a mixture of weedkillers – the chemicals isoproturon and pendimehalin – together with a pyrethroid insecticide, Lambda-cyhalothrin.

The following spring – at the start of stem growth – they're sprayed with a mixture containing two fungicides – propiconazole and Chlorothalonil – to keep the plants free of fungal diseases. Also in the spray mix is a plant growth hormone called Chlormequat; the chemical companies prefer to refer to these compounds as growth 'regulators'.

As the plants grow taller they're sprayed with a further fungicide mixture, this time containing the chemicals Azoxystrobin, Chlorothalonil again, and tetraconazole. Along with the fungicides is a blend of growth hormones – Trinexapac-ethyl, Chlormequat again, choline chloride and iazaquin.

During the stage of rapid stem growth another trio of fungicides are applied – tebuconazole, a second dose of Azoxystrobin and a third close of Chlorothalonil. A final dose of fungicide – metconazole – is sprayed on as the flag leaf emerges. It's this large leaf at the top of the stem that will supply much of the carbohydrate to fill the swelling grains. If it's smothered in fungal disease, the pesticide specialists warn, the final grain yield will be much reduced.

While the wheat plants are being bombarded with agrochemicals they're also receiving large amounts of chemical fertilizer, particularly nitrogen. It's the lush, 'watery' foliage stimulated by the chemical nitrogen that makes the plant susceptible to disease. Hence the need for an endless sequence of fungicide sprays. It's great business for the chemical companies.

This is the kind of spray programme that's followed by thousands of farmers in Britain. The cost in seed and chemicals adds up to about £100 an acre – at 2006 prices, the value of about a ton-and-a-quarter of wheat. Without subsidies most farmers would never have grown crops this way.

The Cereals Event is a show dedicated to the hard-headed, grown-up business of driving down production costs and maximizing profits. To see this in action I headed for the wide arable plains of Lincolnshire.

I followed the signs and parked in the show carpark – one enormous field. Away in the distance a small township of marquees, awnings, banners and flags had sprung up in the middle of an arable prairie. It was as if the army of Gengis Khan had pitched camp on the vast, open steppes.

I took a stroll among the crowded trade stands. The year's crop of gleaming new farm machines looked bigger than ever. There were giant combine harvesters capable of swallowing up dozens of acres of wheat in a single day, and ranks of heavy-duty cultivators ready to stir up and shatter the soil in preparation for the next crop.

New crop varieties were much in evidence, too. The plant breeding companies are constantly introducing new wheats that promise just a little more yield or better bread-making qualities. The new high performers have names like Einstein, Gladiator, Smuggler and Nijinsky.

But the real stars of the Big Wheat Fest are chemicals – the fertilizers and pesticides that underpin crop growing across the western world. Most of the demonstration plots are devoted to them. And the largest, plushest trade stands belong to the companies that market them.

There was even a demonstration arena devoted to spraying machines. No fewer than 39 sprayers would be put through their paces, the show programme promised.

Farm chemicals and the marketing of them are the reasons for this great rural jamboree. And in the wider world they're the reasons why we grow our crops in the way we do.

I joined a small group of farmers walking around the demonstration plots – small-scale wheat crops grown to show off a new variety or the effects of the latest fungicide. Beside one plot of dense, weed-free plants there was a sign listing all the chemicals that had gone on them.

That's what the go-ahead farmer of the twenty-first century puts on the wheat that will go into our 'healthy' breakfast cereals or the 'nourishing' daily loaf.

I turned to a farmer standing next to me. He was wearing a bright check shirt and a baseball cap bearing the logo of an American tractor company.

'Just think what you'd save if you didn't use any of this stuff,' I said in a jocular sort of way. He looked at me as if I needed sectioning under the Mental Health Act.

'If you didn't use 'em you wouldn't get a bloody crop at all,' he muttered, and walked off to inspect the new varieties.

As it happens he was wrong. Wheat was feeding entire civilizations thousands of years before fungicides were dreamt of. This was the grain found in earthenware jars by archaeologists opening up the tombs of the Egyptian pharaohs. In ancient Greece, Hippocrates, the father of medicine, recommended stone-ground flour for its beneficial effects on the digestion.

When I first got interested in farming in the mid-1960s, wheat was grown by what would today be called low-input methods. The farmer I worked for grew mostly spring-sown varieties. The place wasn't entirely chemical-free: a little nitrogen fertilizer went 'down the spout' with the seed when it was drilled in March.

But once the crop had been sown and rolled in there wasn't much else to do. In those days there were no fungicides to protect against disease. Nor were they needed. The farmer simply shut the gate and walked away until harvest time, apart from the occasional visit to see how the crop was progressing.

Yields varied, of course, just as they do now. In a good year we might harvest two- or two-and-a-half tons of grain to the acre. Today yields are more than twice as big. But there's far less profit in it for the farmer. The extra income is swallowed up in the cost of chemicals. And at the end of it consumers get a degraded product.

Residues from pesticides (a term commonly used to describe all crop chemicals) turn up routinely in today's bread. In 2003, 56 out of 72 samples tested by the UK Pesticide Residues Committee – the government's official watchdog – were found to be contaminated.[1] The four most common contaminants were Chlormequat, the growth hormone; glyphosate, a non-selective weedkiller; malathion and pirimphos-methyl, both insecticides.

The three chemicals found at the highest levels in bread were subjected to risk assessments by the residues committee. They concluded that 'there was no concern for human health'. Not all experts agree.

The weedkiller glyphosate – which is widely used in the production of wheat and other crops – is marketed by its manufacturers as largely benign. They describe the pesticide products containing the chemical as of 'low toxicity'. In fact these products are acutely toxic to animals, including human beings. The symptoms include eye and skin irritation, headache, nausea, numbness, raised blood pressure and heart palpitations.[2]

In California, studies on occupational risks showed glyphosate-containing weedkillers to be the third most commonly-reported cause of pesticide illness among agricultural workers.[3] While many of the reports concerned 'irritant effects', mostly to the eyes and skin, a survey of one hundred reports found that over half of them involved more serious effects, including burning of eyes or skin, blurred vision, skin peeling, nausea, headache, vomiting, diarrhoea, chest pain, dizziness, numbness, burning of the genitals and wheezing.[4]

Exposure to malathion – an organo-phosphate insecticide – produces a range of symptoms, including headache, nausea, burning eyes and breathing difficulties.[5] In laboratory studies it has given rise to genetic changes in mice. According to the United States Environmental Protection Agency, there is 'suggestive evidence' that the chemical causes cancer.[6] Later studies have provided firmer evidence. A commercial malathion insecticide product caused breast cancer in laboratory animals.[7]

The government's so-called risk assessment is a desk study taking account of the known toxicity of a chemical compound and the theoretical intake of people eating the bread. It pretty well rules out any catastrophic, short-term threat to health. No one's going to collapse after eating from a contaminated loaf. But it cannot measure the long-term risk of consuming small amounts of different chemicals over many years.

Yet this is the kind of chemical cocktail consumed daily by almost everyone who eats non-organic bread. Current safety tests are carried out on each chemical in isolation. But there's evidence that a combination of two or three pesticides at low levels can be many times more harmful than the individual chemicals acting alone.

Dr Vyvyan Howard, a pathologist specializing in the effect of toxins on human development, says a true test of pesticide safety would mean testing them in all possible combinations. Since this would be impossible, it makes sense to minimize human exposure to these chemicals.[8]

In Canada, the Ontario College of Family Physicians – a voluntary, non-profit making association of doctors – has carried out a comprehensive review of research into pesticide hazards. As a result, they have recommended that people reduce their exposure to these chemicals 'wherever possible'.[9]

In their study, the Canadian doctors found 'positive associations' between pesticide exposure and a number of cancers, including those of the brain, prostate, kidney and pancreas. They also discovered a 'remarkable consistency' in research linking pesticide exposure to damage of the nervous system.

Occupational exposure to agrochemicals might also be associated with reproductive damage, including birth defects, foetal death and retarded growth in the uterus.

Dr Margaret Sanborn, one of the report's authors, concluded: 'Many of the health problems linked with pesticide use are serious and difficult to treat. So we are advocating reducing exposure to pesticides and prevention of harm as the best approach.'

But it's not pesticide contamination alone that has spoiled this everyday food. The battery of chemicals used in the growing of wheat also robs it of the vitamins and minerals that once made it so healthy (see box on page 72).

As mentioned earlier, on the Thames Valley farm where I worked in the 1960s, crops were still sown into fertile soils – soils enriched by plant and animal residues from the grass 'ley' that always preceded wheat. As the land warmed up in spring, soil micro-organisms got to work on these residues, breaking them down and releasing minerals in the form plants could use them.

Organisms called mycorrhiza flourished in these soils, helping crops extract the nutrients they needed. Wheat plants generally stayed healthy without the need for fungicide sprays. The natural living processes of the soil produced the conditions in which they could thrive.

Forty years on, that system of farming looks as ancient as the bullock cart. Modern wheat growing is chiefly a matter of selecting the appropriate chemicals and spraying them on at the right time. Today's wheat crops receive, on average, three doses of weedkiller, three fungicides, a growth regulator and an insecticide.

The transformation came with the introduction of 'tramlines'. These are the regularly-spaced wheel marks that allow the farmer to go on spraying throughout the growing season. Since farmers are now able to spray fungicides whenever they choose, they put on far more chemical fertilizers than they used to. If the extra dose of chemical nitrogen threatens to knock the crop down, they simply go in with the sprayer and give it a shot of growth hormone to stiffen it up. And when the fertilizer leads to more disease in the crop, there's a remedy at hand – an extra spray of fungicide.

Today there's scarcely a wheat crop in the land that doesn't have the telltale wheel-marks running through it. And there's hardly a month of the year – from early autumn to high summer – when you're not guaranteed to see a tractor and sprayer trundling along them.

So profligate are wheat growers with their chemicals that they're producing new super-races of weeds and diseases. Weedkiller-resistant forms of blackgrass, wild oats and common chickweed are widespread. So are fungicide-resistant strains of the crop diseases mildew, septoria and yellow rust.

In the face of this threat of their own making, the chemical companies are urging farmers to use yet more chemicals. Their advice is to use a whole range of pesticides all with different modes of action against the target species. They make it easy by supplying ready-made chemical mixtures to fox the bugs.

What no one suggests is a return to growing crops on fertile soils. The countryside is now run by a generation of farmers who are convinced that chemical agriculture is the only way to grow crops for profit. But the chemical onslaught didn't come about because of some immutable law of progress. It is a legacy of political mismanagement. And it was largely funded by the taxpayer.

In 1973 when Britain joined the European Economic Community – the Common Market as it was – we became bound by the rules and regulations of the Common Agricultural Policy. Farmers were at once paid inflated prices for most agricultural products. For wheat, this artificial market was supported by border taxes on imports and generous subsidies on exports, allowing European surpluses to be dumped on world markets.

In this protected climate, farmers could afford to ditch their time-honoured practice of mixed farming. One of the benefits of having both livestock and cash crops on the farm was that it provided a measure of protection against a fall in the price of any particular commodity.

When the wheat price tumbled there were always sales of milk, beef or lamb to offset the loss. And when the price of

The link between soil fertility and the health of the crop is far from new. It's an idea developed by a scientist working a century ago. Sir Albert Howard spent much of his early career in India, eventually becoming director of the Institute of Plant Industry in the state of Indore. One of his first jobs in the country was to improve crops growing on the research station at Pusa in Bengal.

He soon discovered there wasn't much he could teach the locals about good food. He was struck immediately by the vibrant health of the crops grown by Bengali farmers. He decided to try out their methods on the crops grown at the research station.

As he became more skilled so the incidence of crop disease steadily fell. Within a few years he had learned how to grow healthy, disease-free crops. He was convinced that fertile soils – rich in humus from the breakdown of plant and animal wastes – were essential for the growing of healthy foods. He later wrote that plants were nourished in two ways.[10] First they absorbed through their roots small quantities of nitrate, phosphate and potash salts from solution in the soil. But they also relied on the symbiotic relationship with mycorrhizal fungi for many other nutrients.

Only when plants were nourished in this double way were they able to take up adequate levels of trace elements. And only then could they resist disease and produce high-quality foods for both animals and human beings, noted Howard.

In marked contrast, crops grown with chemical fertilizers were only partially nourished. Chemical farming destroyed soil humus and severed the link with mycorrhiza. Crop plants were no longer resistant to disease. Nor were their products able to protect human health as well as foods from well-nourished plants.

More than sixty years after Howard issued his dire warning, it is now largely forgotten.

lamb or beef was low, the chances were that cereal prices would be on the way up. 'Down horn, up corn' went the old farming adage.

With high prices guaranteed by Brussels, farmers no longer needed a range of different enterprises to give them financial stability. Looking after animals every day of the year was demanding, so many chose to get rid of their livestock and re-invent themselves as specialist wheat growers.

It was likely to be costly in machinery and chemicals. And without cattle and sheep to maintain fertility, plant nutrients would have to be bought in as fertilizers. That's why the UK wheat area has doubled to five million acres since 1973.[11]

In this new super-heated farm economy, the chemical companies have been quick to seize their opportunity. In this they were ably assisted by the plant breeders who have delivered a host of varieties that need chemicals to thrive.

In the mid-twentieth century in Mexico, Norman Borlaug developed a clutch of short-strawed wheats from a Japanese variety. It was a breeding programme that would lead to the Green Revolution and win him the Nobel Peace Prize (see page 169). Some of the new breeding material was crossed with a variety called Cappelle Desprez, a wheat that was once widely-grown in Britain. From this cross a team at Cambridge developed a family of semi-dwarf varieties, the first of which was called Hobbit.

These new short-strawed wheats had a greatly improved 'standing power' – they were far less likely to lodge (i.e. fall over). This meant the farmer could safely put on far higher levels of nitrogen fertilizer without the risk of damage.

Compared with traditional tall wheats, the short-strawed varieties directed a higher proportion of sugars into the seed-head, the 'ear' of the plant. In this way they were capable of producing dramatically higher yields, but to achieve it they needed high inputs of chemical nitrogen. At a stroke an ancient grain had been made a hostage to the multinational chemical industry.

'Thirty years of progress', says the headline above a special feature in the weekly farming tabloid *Farmers Guardian*. The feature – sponsored by Monsanto, makers of the top-selling weedkiller Roundup – celebrates the wheat-growing revolution that has marked Britain's three decades of membership of the European Community.

It is a revolution that has brought few benefits for consumers. In a generation it has demolished the safe and stable pattern of mixed farming that delivered wholesome, nutrient-rich grain. It has given them instead wasteful surpluses of a degraded product, depleted of nutrients and laced with pesticide residues.

It's a system of farming that has its origins on the other side of the Atlantic – in the heartland of the United States. Modern intensive wheat production was nurtured by white settlers on the vast American prairies.

Wheat growing is part of the American dream. As Americans began to populate the vast territory west of the Mississippi – the lands that had been acquired from France in the early nineteenth century – the 'wilderness' at America's heart became productive through the hard work and fortitude of the homesteaders. That is the legend.

In reality, this land wasn't a wilderness at all. It was a highly productive, grassland ecosystem supporting a wealth of life forms. For a brief period, the Europeans respected this living producer of plenty.

From the mid-nineteenth century, the white settlers began to destroy the great natural production system. They ripped up the ancient turf with their steel ploughs and planted the new Turkey Red wheat, which was tough enough to withstand the harsh prairie climate.

For a few decades they harvested bumper crops, nourished as they were by a thousand years of accumulated fertility. Grain poured from these untouched soils and was exported across the world, bringing ruin to many a British farmer.

By the 1930s, it was all over. The prairies died in a billowing, black dust cloud that rolled across the nation's heartland turning day into night. Robbed of its life-giving organic matter, the soil simply blew away in the Dust Bowl of the West.

Today, the prairie-lands still grow crops – mostly corn,

wheat and soya – but only because they are constantly dosed with chemical fertilizers and pesticides, and because the US government is prepared to spend billions of dollars annually on irrigation and subsidies. Two-thirds of the grain is then fed to the cattle that have replaced the bison slaughtered by the settlers.

American grain growing is the enemy of traditional agriculture. It is an extractive industry, a mining of the soil; an exploitation of an ancient storehouse of fertility using industrial tools – hybrid seeds, pesticides and fertilizers. It's also a 'lame-duck industry', wholly dependent on public subsidies for its continuing survival. Yet this is the model of grain growing that America has exported to the world.

A handful of food grains – wheat, maize and rice – produced this way now dominates world diets. Their production relies on huge inputs of fertilizer and pesticides, generating big profits for the chemical companies and machinery manufacturers.

No doubt the 'miracle seeds' – the compact, fertilizer-dependent crop varieties of the 1960s and 1970s – fed millions who might otherwise have gone hungry. But they could have been fed far better.

A United Nations report estimates that two billion people around the world now suffer from 'hidden hunger' – vitamin and mineral deficiencies that undermine their physical and mental health.

The essential nutrients that have fallen to critically low levels include iron, zinc, iodine, vitamin A and folic acid. As a remedy, the UN is proposing a whole range of 'fortified foods', such as soy sauce with added zinc, salt with extra iron and cooking oil fortified with vitamin A.

Modern chemical wheat production is designed to produce surpluses and drive down prices. Under its ruthless rules only the biggest farmers can make a profit, while small farmers and farmworkers are driven from the land.

In Britain, 'big wheat' has cost the jobs of thousands of farm staff as farms have grown bigger and their owners have relied on large machines. It's the advance of intensive wheat growing that has pushed families from the countryside, emptying village schools and closing village shops. And the devastation continues because consumers are willing to put up with degraded food.

The capacity of the 'big wheat' industry to put small farmers out of business has been described as a kind of 'warfare' by Vandana Shiva, who trained as a quantum physicist but now campaigns for traditional farming in her native India. Industrial agriculture, she says, has become a war against

---

The alternative approach to grain growing has been demonstrated by Takao Furuno, a farmer in southern Japan, and author of *The Power of Duck*. He was determined not to grow rice in a conventional monoculture, with its dependence on pesticides and fertilizers. Instead of the industrial paradigm he took an ecological approach, introducing fish and ducks into his paddy fields.

First he planted his rice seedlings into the flooded paddies. He then introduced a gaggle of ducklings, which started feeding on the insects that would normally attack young rice plants. Next he brought in loaches, an edible fish that is easily cultivated and produces tasty meat. He also planted azolla, a nitrogen-fixing herb that's usually thought of as a weed.

In Furuno's paddy fields the ducks feed on insects, and – like the loaches – on the azolla weed. Since it is continuously grazed the weed never becomes dominant enough to compete with the rice. At the same time it supplies nitrogen to the crop. Add this to the droppings from the ducks and fish, and the rice gets all the nutrients it needs.

Around his paddy fields Furuno has integrated vegetable, wheat and fig crops. Without fertilizers or pesticides he harvests rice crops that are up to half as big again as industrial rice-growing systems. His six-acre farm produces a gross income slightly higher than the average six-hundred-acre rice farm in Texas.[13]

ecosystems.[12] It is based on the instruments of war – chemicals originally made for chemical warfare – and the logic of war, based on ideas of dominance and the destruction of diversity.

She challenges the 'myth' that the industrial growing of grains is more productive than traditional, ecological agriculture based on a range of different crops. Traditional farming systems evolved because more food could be harvested from an area planted with a mixture of crops than from the same area growing separate patches of monoculture.

The ecological approach to high-yield farming of rice (as undertaken by Takao Furuno, see page 76) can be applied equally well to wheat. French ecologist and farmer Marc Bonfils developed a system of wheat growing that produced spectacular yields without fertilizers or pesticides.[14] Instead he made full use of the strength and vigour of the ancient wheat plant before it was weakened by modern plant breeders trying to shorten the straw. He also utilized the natural fertility-building power of clover plants to provide the nutrients – particularly nitrates – for a healthy grain crop.

Today's wheat growers plant their hybrid seeds in early autumn for harvesting in summer the following year. They have to sow the seeds densely. Soil temperatures will soon begin to fall and widely-spaced plants wouldn't have time to develop a thick crop before the onset of winter.

By the time the frosts come modern crops are still struggling to put down decent root systems. That's why large amounts of chemical nitrogen have to be applied the following spring if the still-frail crop is to produce a decent harvest. And because spring growth is 'forced' with nitrogen fertilizer, the plants must be bombarded with pesticides to keep them alive.

Marc Bonfils took a radically different approach. He discovered, through research, that ancient wheat varieties were remarkably strong and robust. They had the capacity to grow dozens of side shoots producing wheat 'bushes' instead of the single stems that characterize chemically-grown crops. These bushes were able to put down huge root systems, but to do so they had to be planted far earlier in the year.

On the Bonfils system, winter wheat is sown in early summer

– just a few days after the solstice in June. By the start of winter the plants have developed numerous side shoots and extensive root systems. When the soil warms up in the following spring they're ready to throw up masses of seed-heads.

In another radical feature, the seeds are sown into a low-growing clover crop. It's the natural action of soil microbes at the clover roots that produces the nitrogen the growing wheat plants need. Well-nourished in a fertile soil the crop stays healthy without the need for pesticides. And at harvest – which is two weeks earlier than for chemically-grown crops – it produces a bigger yield than the modern dwarf hybrids.

The Bonfils system is ignored by the farming establishment. Not surprisingly the agrochemical manufacturers – who dominate the industry – see it as a threat. Developed on a larger scale it could provide health-giving wheat grains, free of pesticide residues and rich in essential vitamins and minerals. But this isn't likely to happen.

Impoverished foods have long been the legacy of chemical wheat growing. Around the time the American homesteaders were ripping up the prairie grassland, a parallel revolution was taking place in the flour milling business. A group of commercial millers in Minnesota installed a new French device called the purifier, which separated flour from the coarser parts of the grain.

This was quickly followed by the roller-mill, a high-speed machine in which the traditional millstones were replaced with steel rollers. Within two decades the new milling process had made the old-style gristmill obsolete. The business of milling was transformed from a small-scale local enterprise to a factory process turning out thousands of tons of white flour.

In Britain, the new-style mills were built at ports so they could process imported American wheat. Until then the local gristmill had been a key part of the rural economy. Almost overnight they were made uneconomic. Milling had become an industrial process. The local baker – obtaining his flour from the country mill – was replaced by the 'plant baker', the large-scale manufacturer of white bread.

A century ago, the writer William Edgar hailed the milling

revolution as a great advance for civilization. In *The Story of a Grain of Wheat* he celebrates the close of 'the era of black bread, coarse and dirty, fit only for strong teeth and the digestive apparatus of a rugged outdoor man.' Gone, at last, were 'the black bread times, when the flour of all save the very rich was dark and filled with impurities.'[15]

The belief that white bread was somehow superior has become a dominant idea in the industrial world. The wrestlers and athletes of ancient Greece may have insisted on coarse wheat bread to maintain their power and strength. But in the modern world we're all convinced that white flour is a far finer food.

When wheat was ground between stones in traditional gristmills, the flour retained all the nutrients of the original grain. Modern roller-mills reject all but the starchy endosperm of the grain. The bran and wheat germ are lost, along with many of the minerals, vitamins and essential fatty acids.

The resulting white flour contains only a small fraction of the original nutrients. To compensate, the plant bakers are required to 'enrich' or 'fortify' white bread with a number of added nutrients. It's hardly an equal trade.

During processing, millers remove up to 80 per cent of the nutrients in the original grain. These include the minerals calcium, zinc, copper, iron, magnesium, manganese, potassium, phosphorus and selenium; the B vitamins niacin, riboflavin, thiamine and pyridoxin; and vitamin E. In return the millers add calcium, iron, thiamine and niacin.

When bread and everyday wheat products have been degraded by fortification (see page 80) it's hardly surprising the wheat growers pay scant attention to the nutrient content of their crop. They no longer grow a food. Instead they are producing a raw material for an industrial manufacturing operation.

So long as they can meet the technical demands of the plant bakers, farmers have only one concern – the size of their harvest. Grain yield per acre becomes an obsession – a badge of achievement, a mark of status. This is why they will push fertilizers and sprays to the limit. They must squeeze ever more production from their over-worked soils.

In her book *Nourishing Traditions*, nutritionist Sally Fallon debunks the idea of 'fortification'.[16] It adds a handful of synthetic vitamins and minerals to white flour after dozens of essential nutrients have been removed or destroyed. Some of the added nutrients may even be harmful. There's evidence that excess iron from fortified flour can cause tissue damage, and other studies link excess or toxic iron to heart disease. Vitamins B1 and B2 – added to grains without vitamin B6 – lead to imbalances in numerous processes involving B vitamin pathways.

Fallon is no more enthusiastic about the treatment of grains that go into modern breakfast cereals. She writes, 'Whole grains that have been processed by high heat and pressure to produce puffed wheat, oats and rice are actually quite toxic and have caused rapid death in test animals. Breakfast cereals that have been slurried and extruded at high temperatures and pressures to make little flakes and shapes should also be avoided. Most, if not all, nutrients are destroyed during processing, and they are very difficult to digest. Studies show that these extruded whole grain preparations can have even more adverse effects on the blood sugar that refined sugar and white flour.'

Vast amounts of chemically-grown wheat now swirl around the world wreaking havoc with local food systems. It matters little whether the grain is grown on the American plains, the Paris basin or in Lincolnshire – the results are the same. Markets for wholesome, traditional foods are undermined and sustainable farms are put out of business.

Chief beneficiaries are the oil and chemical companies, global commodity traders and the large-scale livestock farmers, who take their animals off pasture where they belong and feed them the unhealthy grain. In this way commodity grain degrades the general food supply.

Fortunately, this way of farming is unlikely to survive for much longer. US agrarian writer Gene Logsdon expects large-scale industrial wheat-growing to collapse under its crippling burden of costs – those of the fertilizers, pesticides and machinery needed to keep the grain flowing.[17] Instead the western world will come to rely on 'pasture farming' for its food, with grazing animals providing meat, milk, eggs, dairy products, wool and hundreds of other animal products, at a fraction of the cost of producing them with current factory technology. Logsdon says:

> Pasture farming is the first alternative to high-tech agriculture that has both short-term and long-term profit on its side. Industrial grain farming and animal factories may have had short-term profit advantage for a while. That's why they rose to prominence, but no longer. Over half the money to keep these operations afloat now comes from government subsidies.
>
> If there is any lesson of history that always remains true, it is that no economy can be falsely sustained when it can't compete with another economy. Neither all the king's horses nor all the king's men can make industrial farming survive with subsidies, just as fifty years of subsidies could not save the old family farm. Industrial farming is simply not profitable enough any more to compete with pasture farming.

6
Pasture-fed Beef

Jim and Kay Barnard raise beef cattle in Somerset. Through the summer months they graze them on the Pawlett Hams, a stretch of flat, low-lying grassland bordering the River Parrett, close to where it runs into the Bristol Channel.

It's an empty, wind-swept sort of place. On a misty morning it's not hard to imagine the Kent marshes where Pip had his first frightening encounter with the convict Magwich in *Great Expectations*.

For centuries the Pawlett Hams have been renowned for producing tasty, succulent beef – the kind of beef the wealthy merchants of Bristol would willingly pay over the odds for. The reason is these lush grasslands were kept fertile and productive by periodic flooding.

Every so often a combination of strong winds and a high tide in the Bristol Channel would send the banked up waters of the estuary cascading over the flood defences. When the flood-waters finally drained away the turf was left covered in dark sediment – a thick, brown cake rich in trace elements from the sea and from the distant Quantock Hills. Mixed with them were organic wastes and detritus from the upstream towns of Langport and Bridgwater.

Over the following seasons the grasses would grow thick on their newly-enriched soils. And the cattle that grazed across them under the summer sun would grow strong and healthy.

It's now more than twenty years since the Hams experienced a serious inundation. The flood defences are better than they used to be. But the Barnards are convinced they are still reaping the benefits in the health and vigour of their livestock.

On a bright November morning, I joined a scratch team of volunteer drovers to help bring the free-ranging cattle in for the winter. In all there were more than 200 beasts to round up and drive back to the yard – the cows and their spring-born calves, now six or seven months old.

We, the drovers, were all of 'a certain age'. The joints were starting to seize up and our stamina wasn't what it used to be. The animals – by contrast – were fit and frisky after a summer and autumn on the open grassland. To reach the yard and buildings we would be herding them along a village lane past half a dozen executive homes – some with pony paddocks – not to mention the village school and playing field. It was going to be an interesting roundup.

Down on the Hams Jim began calling up his livestock. 'C'mon, c'mon, c'mon,' he yelled. The sound spread across the open grassland like floodwater from a broken dyke. The cattle – in anticipation of a succulent bale of silage – bellowed back. From all directions they began converging on us as we climbed down from the tractor and trailer.

As they came close the cows kicked up their heels and ran around us like youngsters. In the general excitement some squared up to each other, lowering their heads in a ritual tussle. The calves looked bewildered at it all.

With much whistling and waving of arms, we managed to get the herd on the move. Bob, the herdsman, led the procession, driving slowly ahead on the tractor. The trailer with its half load of hay bales provided the enticement. Still bellowing wildly the beasts followed across the open grassland while we did our best to discourage any breakaway movements.

After a dry summer the turf still felt firm beneath our feet. In Britain, mid-November is late to be taking cattle off pastureland. On most grass fields the pressure of hoofs would by now have started poaching up the turf. But this stretch of pastureland on a Somerset flood plain wasn't like most grass fields.

For the past thirty years or so, farmers have sown most grass fields with a single species: perennial ryegrass. They've been persuaded by government advisors and the chemical industry that by growing a monoculture and plastering it with large amounts of nitrogen fertilizer, they'll grow more grass to the acre. The chemical companies love perennial ryegrass. It's aggressive and competitive, quickly crowding out other grasses and herbs, particularly in the presence of chemical fertilizer. It's the Darth Vader of the grass kingdom.

But while the fertilized ryegrass monoculture may produce large amounts of leaf tissue, it's not particularly healthy for grazing animals. Sir Albert Howard, the early pioneer of organic farming (see page 72), once referred to it as 'a bastard structure'. It's a kind of ruminant 'fast food', unbalanced in its mineral content. It does little for the health of the animals grazing it, and all too often it wrecks the soil it's grown on.

A few weeks before the roundup on the Hams, I'd seen just such a ruined pasture on a farm in Devon. It was owned by an intensive dairy farmer who had decided to get out of milk. In company with a hundred or so would-be buyers, I tramped the fields on the day the cows were to be sold.

I spotted the damaged grass straight away. The field looked like a replica of a First World War battlefield. Much of it was a sea of mud though there hadn't been any torrential rains in the days leading up to the sale. I sloshed across it in my wellies.

Over large parts of it the grass had all but disappeared. Here and there it survived like small green islands in a choppy brown ocean. This was a field that had been sown with the wrong kind of grass and spread with too much fertilizer.

The turf on the Pawlett Hams could hardly have been more different. Even in mid-November it appeared an unbroken green. This was no monoculture. As we herded the bellowing beasts across it I noticed there were dozens of different plant species.

Some of the agricultural grasses I recognized from my student days: deep-rooting cocksfoot with its ability to stay productive both in wet conditions and in dry; rough-stalked meadow grass; the drought-resistant crested dogs-tail; and the fragrant sweet vernal grass. There was plenty of clover present, both as red-flowering and white varieties. Perennial ryegrass was present in small amounts, but in the absence of nitrogen fertilizer it was never going to become rampant.

My friends once commissioned a botanical survey of their section of the Hams. In all there were found to be thirty-three plant species growing on this small area of flood plain. Along with the grasses many herb species flourished. Had we been here in summer we'd have seen blue forget-me-not, the tiny white flowers of mouse-ear, tall lady's smock with its blush-pink blooms, and bright red pimpernel.

Over the years these low-lying pastures have received scarcely any fertilizers and no pesticide sprays. There's every possibility that these same species were seen by the farmers and graziers of Tudor England when they turned out their cattle. The fact that they have survived over the centuries isn't simply of interest to botanists. It's the reason why cattle grazing here remain so fit and healthy. And it's why the beef they produced was valued for its taste and succulence as well as for its health-giving properties.

By the time we'd got our 200 charges as far as the village lane, their vitality was beginning to tell on the ageing drovers. They'd been relatively easy to coax across the open grassland of the Hams. The powerful herd instinct had kept them together and moving in roughly the right direction. But as they funnelled through the narrow gateway leading into the village lane the social cohesion began to break down.

Pressed into a narrow thoroughfare between flimsy fences and hedges, the bellowing herd were soon strung out over two hundred metres or so. No longer did the dominant cows at the head of the procession dictate the direction of movement. At almost any point along the line an independent-minded beast was liable to make a dash towards a well-manicured lawn or a well-stocked flower border.

We did our best to anticipate such breakaway movements, slamming shut garden gates and standing in driveways gesticulating wildly. Finally, breathless and exhausted, we managed to herd the stragglers through the yard gate. At that point the cattle looked in a lot better shape than we were.

'That's what happens down on the Hams,' said Jim, recovering his breath. 'They always do well on that old grassland – everything does. I've never seen cattle put on weight so fast.'

A few years earlier Jim and Kay had been dairy farmers. As is standard practice in modern dairy herds they routinely took calves from their mothers at just a few days old. Milk was far too valuable to waste on the infant animals nature had intended it for. Artificial milk substitute was quite good enough for them.

Jim recalls that calves reared in this unnatural way grew at barely half the rate of these young beef animals, which had spent the summer with their mothers on old, mixed pasture. At six or seven months old, these youngsters were grazing on a mineral-rich turf while still suckling from their mothers.

Ironically, most modern farmers – weaned on the chemical habit – would consider such ancient grazings hopelessly unproductive. The conventional view of a profitable grass field is one sown to perennial ryegrass and plastered with ammonium nitrate fertilizer. It's a notion that has done untold harm to livestock and robbed consumers of the chance to eat healthy meat and dairy products.

Modern grass monocultures are poor at harvesting essential trace elements from the soil. With only a single species of grass present, roots penetrate to the same depth in the soil. The only minerals they are able to take up are those available at this one level in the soil 'horizon'. By contrast, species-rich pastures – such as those on the Pawlett Hams – have a variety of root systems growing to different depths. So they can take up minerals from various levels in the soil and concentrate them in the herbage where grazing livestock can make the most of them.

Traditional mixed grasslands contained a wide range of plant species, some of them grasses, some of them herbs. Each species would have its own distinct mineral 'profile' – an assembly of chemical elements that was unique to the plant. With a diverse 'community' of plants making up the pasture, livestock were able to graze selectively, choosing the plants that would provide them with optimum nutrition.

This was the natural order of things – the system produced by evolution to ensure healthy animals and sustainable grasslands. Until the arrival of cheap nitrate fertilizer, no self-respecting livestock farmer would have dreamt of sowing a new pasture, or ley, without including at least half a dozen different species in the seeds mixture. Diversity was seen as essential to the proper nutrition of the grazing animal. There would be, perhaps, two or three grass species along with at least one sort of clover to provide protein and minerals, and to boost soil fertility by fixing atmospheric nitrogen at the root nodules.

Some farmers went a great deal further. But the warnings of these traditional farmers went unheeded. Today nitrate fertilizers have changed Britain's pastures beyond recognition. They have destroyed the grassland herbs and delivered up the fields to perennial ryegrass.

No longer can cattle graze on a pasture well-endowed with minerals and vitamins. In an attempt to compensate, many stock farmers now provide mineral blocks for their animals to lick. But like mineral supplements for humans, these 'licks' are no substitute for a proper level of trace elements in food. To be metabolized efficiently, most minerals must be accompanied by a range of other nutrients. It's the full assembly – found together in well-grown natural foods – that provides sound nutrition.

The grasses now fed to cattle have all the mineral content of over-boiled cabbage. As a result, consumers are supplied with sub-standard meat. No longer does it contain the full complement of minerals found in beef before the chemical age.

Raised naturally on fertile soil, beef could be one of the healthiest foods available. Red meat provides complete protein, including sulphur-containing amino acids like cysteine. Beef is a rich source of taurine and carnitine. Both are needed for healthy eyes and a sound heart. It's also rich in co-enzyme Q10, which is important for the cardiovascular system.

Properly reared beef ought to be well-endowed with minerals, including zinc, the prerequisite of clear thought and an

In Somerset, Newman Turner – author of the 1950s classic *Fertility Farming* – included more than twenty different species in the seeds mixture of every new grass ley he sowed.[1] Among them were nine varieties of agricultural grass and four types of clover, both red-flowering and white. The rest were herb species such as chicory, burnet, yarrow, sheep's parsley, kidney vetch, lucerne and plantain. Even seeds of the much-reviled dandelion were included.

In this book, telling the story of Goosegreen, his farm near Bridgwater, Turner wrote: 'A mixture containing deep-rooted herbs is essential to soil, crop and animal health, assisting in the aeration of the subsoil and the transfer from subsoil to topsoil of essential minerals and trace elements.

'Especially important are herbs like chicory, burnet, lucerne and dandelion, all of which penetrate to a depth of three or four feet or more in as many years.'

Turner shunned chemical fertilizers and pesticides. Having relied on them early in his farming career he had become convinced they were damaging to his livestock and ruinous of his land. Instead he came to depend on organic compost and herb-rich pastures for bumper crops and healthy cattle. And they proved to be remarkably successful at the job.

He claimed that by providing his cattle with organically-grown, mineral-rich pasture he was able to prevent, and even cure, many of the most crippling animal afflictions, including TB, infertility, mastitis and Johnes disease – a condition of the intestinal tract like Crohn's disease in humans, and thought to be caused by para-tuberculosis bacteria in milk. Today these diseases remain rife in Britain's cattle population.

So confident was he of his methods that he was known to travel around local markets looking for sick animals, especially those that were clearly suffering from TB. He was confident he could cure them and return them to health and production, so making himself a pound or two.

More than thirty years after his book first appeared, nearly 2,500 British cattle herds are held under TB restrictions.

Farmers blame badgers for the spread of the disease among their stock. They want government action to curb the rising badger population.

To Turner, the argument would have seemed pointless. What did it matter how any disease organism came to be in a particular place? It was the health of an animal's immune system that determined whether or not it contracted the condition. He was convinced it wasn't the TB bacillus that caused disease, but inadequate nutrition. While cattle remain well nourished disease organisms would do them no harm.

In *Fertility Farming*, he tells the story of his favourite stock-bull – a prize-winning Jersey with the colourful name Long-moor Mogulla's Top Sergente. A routine TB test showed the animal to be 'a violent reactor'. The Ministry of Agriculture recommended that it be 'disposed of'.

Turner had different ideas. He isolated the bull on some off-lying land and put him on a carefully-managed diet of fresh, green foods grown on a fertile soil. Meanwhile the Ministry vets continued to test the bull for TB. After a few months they declared he was free of infection. Five years later he was still winning awards and siring prize-winning daughters.

Turner concludes: 'All my work indicates that tuberculosis can be prevented and cured by food grown on a properly-managed soil, provided an adequate ration of mineral-rich herbs is included.'

Half a century before Turner proved the health-giving properties of a species-rich Somerset pasture, a Scottish landowner – named by his neighbours as 'the daft laird' – was carrying out similar experiments in the border country near Kelso. Robert Elliot had made his fortune growing coffee in Mysore in India. With his money he bought the Clifton Estate in Roxburgh-shire, and in 1887 began farming the land at Clifton-on-Beaumont. Until his death in 1914, his chief interest was in species-rich grassland and its capacity to produce fertile soils and healthy livestock.

Like Turner, he believed in using seeds mixtures containing

a variety of deep-rooting herbs. Burnet, chicory, alsike clover and yarrow were the key constituents. Elliot became convinced that not only were herb-rich pastures beneficial to cattle and sheep, but they greatly improved the health of the soil.

Plants like yarrow, vetch, burnet and chicory thrust their roots deep into the ground, breaking up any areas of compaction. As well as drawing minerals and moisture to the surface layers, they opened up the soil, or, in Elliot's terms, 'disintegrated it', so allowing life-giving oxygen to penetrate the deeper levels.

Farmers had no need of chemical fertilizers, he later wrote. The cheapest soil conditioner was a turf made up chiefly of deep-rooting herbs. Plant roots were far-and-away the deepest and best tillers, drainers and warmers of the soil.

In his later years, the old laird took to walking over his best pasture fields 'mending' them with a garden rake and a little bag of seeds. During a wet summer the family coach would arrive early at Clifton Park to drive him and his equipment the four miles to the farm. These little excursions may have been the origin of the 'daft' epithet. But Elliot had a sound message for the farmers of Britain.

At the time he was carrying out his experiments, the country was awash – as now – with cheap food imports. A century ago the competition came from the virgin lands of the Empire – the prairie wheat lands of Canada and the wide, fertile grasslands of New Zealand and South Africa. Britain, the great industrial power, relied on her manufacturing industry to pay for food imports.

Elliot warned that the day would come when countries like China, Japan and India would emerge as powerful industrial nations.[2] To survive in this new competitive world, Britain would have to make use of her most valuable resource – her herb-rich grasslands and their ability to produce strong livestock and health-giving foods.

The constant reliance on artificial fertilizers would cost farmers dear, he warned. In the end it would empty their bank accounts and exhaust the soil.

active sex life. It's also likely to be rich in vitamin B12 – vital for healthy nervous and vascular systems – along with the fat-soluble vitamins A and D.

All these are well-known attributes of beef reared traditionally on fertile pasture. But modern science has uncovered a new benefit. Grass-fed beef is an important provider of essential fats – the polyunsaturated fatty acids. They include CLA (conjugated linoleic acid) together with the longer chain fatty acids EPA (eicosapentaenoic acid) and DHA (docosahexaenoic acid). All are vital to human health.

CLA is highly protective against cancer.[3] It also promotes the build-up of muscle rather than fat tissue. When cattle are raised on fresh pasture alone, their meat and milk contains as much as five times more CLA than the products of animals fed modern, conventional diets.[4] EPA and DHA – which belong to the group known as omega-3 fatty acids – are needed for a number of vital body functions, among them efficient immune and nervous systems.

In ruminant animals, these essential fatty acids are chiefly found, not in storage fats, but in muscle. That makes meat an important source of these nutrients. Along with oily fish – which are often contaminated with heavy metals – beef is a rich source of both EPA and DHA, so long as it is predominantly grass-fed.

In Britain there have been no dust bowls, as happened in America in the early twentieth century. On this side of the Atlantic, the soils are deeper and more stable. But in a less spectacular way our farmers have destroyed their own fertile grasslands as effectively as the American homesteaders, by ploughing up productive pastures and sowing them to the ubiquitous perennial ryegrass. Others were extinguishing their fields chemically by constant applications of nitrate fertilizer. Pastures robbed of their natural mineral balance now threaten the health of animals and human beings alike.

Industrial farming has mounted a second attack on the health-giving properties of British beef. As a farming student in the 1960s, I was once given a glimpse of what was being hailed as a brave new world of food production.

Given the role of fertile grasslands in producing one of mankind's finest foods, it's hard to see why industrial societies have treated them so recklessly. Throughout the western world productive grasslands have been abused and squandered.

Nowhere has the ruin been greater than on the American prairies. Chapter 5 explained how the nineteenth-century homesteaders destroyed the fertile pastures they moved on to – by digging them up and sowing vast fields of wheat – and how their exploitation of the land ended with the great Dust Bowl of the 1930s.

Before the arrival of European settlers, species-rich grasslands stretched in a continuous garment across the North American heartland – from the forest edge in Canada to the Gulf Coast of south-east Texas; from the foothills of the Rockies to the plains of Illinois and western Indiana.

With up to 400 different plant species in a single square metre of turf, these semi-natural grasslands were hugely productive. For thousands of years they supported vast numbers of bison – up to sixty million of them when the great, wandering herds were at their height.

Through drought and storm the grasslands fed them; through blistering hot summers and freezing winters – and all without chemical fertilizers, pesticides, irrigation or any other of the technical aids without which modern farmers say production is impossible.

Like all grassland communities, the prairie plants gathered minerals from deep in the soil and concentrated them in the top few centimetres. Leaves and roots died and decayed, releasing nutrients to be taken up by other plants. Some leaves were grazed by bison or any one of a handful of other grazing animals such as the elk, deer and pronghorn antelope. The grazers built the plant nutrients into their bone and muscle. They left their wastes – and eventually their carcasses – to the unending cycle of decay and re-growth.

Nothing was lost to the system. Nutrients were constantly

recycled through the great living powerhouse of the turf – in the rampant foliage above ground or in the myriad life processes below. It was a truly sustainable system.

The tribes of Native Americans – who hunted the bison – slipped easily into the cycle. From the bison they took meats that were rich in minerals and vitamins, the gift of a fertile soil. And in due time they returned those same elements to the soil and its permanent covering of grass.

French traders bartered with Native Americans for buffalo meat and hides to ship back east to the towns and cities. Out west the cattlemen raised their hardy Texan Longhorns on the grass-draped plains. But with Federal help the railroads began to snake their way across the prairies. With them came the homesteaders and their steel ploughs, ready to plant the acres of wheat that within a few decades would exhaust the land of all it could offer, and turn their dreams to dust.

Barley beef was the agribusiness answer to the threat of over-production – a threat of its own making. The deluge of substandard grain that followed the widespread adoption of chemical fertilizers brought with it the risk of a market collapse. What better way to keep up the grain price than to convert it to meat and sell it on the hoof?

Unfortunately, putting cattle on a diet of cereal grains is dangerous to the animals and to the people who will one day eat the meat. As Chapter 3 pointed out, cattle are ruminants. They are adapted to eating large amounts of fibrous vegetable matter – in a word, grass. The rumen – the first stomach in a ruminant animal – is merely a large fermentation vessel in which micro-organisms get to work on the cellulose in grass, breaking it down into compounds the animal can use in its own metabolism.

Small amounts of grain do little harm. In their natural grazing environment, animals consume grass seed-heads in summer. Cereals are simply highly-bred grasses. But large quantities of grain invariably make cattle ill. The rumen becomes inflamed and its delicate internal ecology is thrown

Early one summer's morning, a group of us 'agrics' piled into two cars and set out on the tedious journey from North Wales to Lincolnshire. Our destination was a large shed on the edge of an arable field – the kind of building that had begun to appear on industrial estates on the outskirts of towns. But this was no factory for manufacturing screws or widgets. This was a factory for making red meat.

We filed inside to where 200 young cattle stood in the half-light. Never in their short lives were these animals to experience the soft tread of a pasture. Instead they were destined to spend their days standing or lying on concrete slats and eating a diet made up mostly of *barley grains*.

The farmer thought it a wonderful development. He guided us round his beef factory with the pride of a developer opening up the show home. In the slanted light we watched the dismal beasts munching their rations.

'It's a fantastic system,' the farmer enthused. 'I can feed this little lot in no time at all. No more messing about with grazing and fencing and all that malarkey. Dead easy, this is. And the best thing of all, the buggers grow like hell. You take it from me – the way of the future, this is.'

into turmoil. The animal develops a kind of chronic acid indigestion. Toxins leak into the bloodstream, damaging the liver and causing a range of conditions from lameness to paralysis.

On too rich a diet the animal will die. But before that happens it's likely to put on flesh at a rapid rate – which is what appeals to farmers. The chances are the beast will be ready for the butcher at a young age, before too many of the health problems have become apparent.

Today, most American beef is fattened on grains. While United States citizens cherish myths of cowboys and the open range, their steaks are raised in feedlots – large-scale meat production factories that may hold tens of thousands of cattle. The animals are moved into the feedlot as well-grown calves or yearlings. They're held in open compounds and fed by highly-automated systems on a ration made up largely of maize and soya meal with added minerals.

It's the same prairie landscape – whose boundless grasslands once raised healthy meat – that now grows grains for the feedlots. With all the costly inputs of fertilizers, pesticides and irrigation, the prairie states – that supported sixty million bison – now produce the corn and soya to fatten an estimated forty-five million beef cattle.

To Richard Manning, American author of *Grassland*, it makes little sense. He says: 'Seventy per cent of the grain crop of American agriculture goes to the livestock that replaced the bison that ate no grains, and one wonders, what is agriculture for?'[5]

This change in the way beef is reared has had damaging effects on the health of Americans. When cattle are moved from pasture to a grain diet in the feedlot, their stores of omega-3 fatty acids including the nutritionally important EPA and DHA – begin to fall. Each day the animal spends in the feedlot reduces the supply of omega-3 fats.[6] Only 40 per cent of Americans are thought to consume enough of these essential nutrients. Twenty per cent have levels so low they cannot be detected.[7]

Feedlots on the American scale are rare in Britain, but the country once famed for its beef still manages to produce its own unhealthy, cereal-fed variety. I met a Somerset dairy farmer who fattened his bull calves like this. He kept them in a shed on a ration of wheat, with soya meal to boost the protein. These were calves whose mothers had been bred as milk factories, so there wasn't too much fat on them. And it's true that filling them with high-energy cereals quickly put the flesh on.

There was just one snag, the farmer told me in all innocence. If these young animals weren't fed precisely the right amount at exactly the right time, they had a tendency to keel over and die.

This came as something of a shock. I suggested that maybe it wasn't a great idea to feed them a diet so unnatural they were likely to drop dead. What was it doing to the quality of the meat, I wondered? The farmer didn't seem concerned. It was simply a matter of being careful, he told me.

I asked him what happened to his finished bulls – the ones that survived, that is. He told me they ended up in the 'economy mince' of a major supermarket chain.

While few UK farmers rear their beef animals entirely in sheds, most beef animals spend a good part of their lives under cover, on rations rich in cereals or other high-energy foods. Traditionally, cattle housed for the winter would be fed on hay or silage together with root crops and a small amount of cereal. Today's intensive beef 'finishers' feed, on average, more than a tonne of high-energy concentrate feed to each beast they fatten.[8]

The aim of feeding them this way is to keep the beast gaining weight fast and so speed the pay-back time to the producer. But the high-energy feeds must be balanced by protein-rich foods that can be equally damaging to the animal. Among the most widely-used is soya meal – the residue remaining from soya beans after the oil has been extracted, first by crushing and then by the use of an industrial solvent. High-protein soya meal is toxic to the animal's liver.

Taking beef cattle off pasture and feeding them on cereal-rich rations has had dire consequences for the nation's health. It has exacerbated a crisis, which, according to Professor Michael Crawford of North London University, is more serious than obesity. It's the sickness caused by an imbalance of essential fats in the national diet.

To remain healthy, human beings need a variety of essential fats, including two types of polyunsaturated fats, the omega-3 and omega-6 fatty acids. It's the proportion of these two fats that's important for health. In a healthy diet, the ratio of omega-6 to omega-3 fats should be no higher than four to one. In the diets of our Stone Age ancestors it was believed to have been in balance.[9] And in the traditional Greek diet – thought to be the healthiest in Europe – the proportion of omega-6 to omega-3 fats is less than two to one.

In most European and American diets, the ratio can be as high as twenty to one. Because of the popularity of cereal foods and oils such as sunflower oil – all of which are rich in omega-6 fats

– the level of dietary omega-3 fat has dropped dramatically.

In the body the two fats act as building blocks for the membranes surrounding neurones, the nerve cells. Omega-3 fatty acids enable the cells to function efficiently. They also help them build links with other neurones, constructing the lattice of nerve connections, which is the basis of intelligence.

The last three months of a pregnancy – and the early weeks in the life of the infant – are critical times for the laying down of this brain cell lattice. To ensure the child's healthy development, the mother must be getting adequate levels of omega-3 fats in her diet. These essential fats are found in vegetables such as cabbage and broccoli. They are also plentiful in fish, and in the meat of cattle grazed on pasture. The rise of factory farming and the transfer of beef cattle from grass to cereal-based diets has steadily eroded an important source of omega-3 fats and contributed to a breakdown in mental and physical health.

Pregnant women on low omega-3 diets are at increased risk of depression.[10] And their children are more likely to suffer from behavioural and co-ordination difficulties. They are also likely to score badly in IQ tests. A number of studies have shown a link between aggressive behaviour in children and low dietary levels of omega-3 fats.[11]

The effects of this fat imbalance continue into adulthood. American researchers have shown that people with low blood levels of omega-3 fats are at a higher risk of heart attack than those with higher levels. Where the level of dietary omega-3s was considered ample, the risk of a serious heart attack was reduced by half.[12]

People whose diets are rich in omega-3s are also less likely to suffer from depression, schizophrenia, hyperactivity or Alzheimer's disease,[13] and they're likely to be at a reduced risk from cancer.[14]

In the light of these findings food scientists are looking at ways of boosting omega-3 fat levels in meat by adding linseed oil to the rations of housed cattle. It's the classic industrial response to a threat caused in the first place by the industrialization of agriculture.

The traditional way to raise beef was to graze cattle on

pasture. By restoring cattle to their natural environment farmers could again ensure that beef made a major contribution to the level of omega-3 fatty acids in the western diet. It would have the added advantage of raising dietary levels of CLA, the polyunsaturated fatty acid that protects against cancer and promotes weight loss.

The decline of beef as a healthy food is reflected in the breeds of cattle that now stock the fields and cattle-yards. In the nineteenth century, British beef cattle were sought around the world. Famous native breeds, such as the Hereford, the Shorthorn, the North Devon, the Aberdeen Angus, the Sussex, the Welsh Black and the Ayrshire, were almost synonymous with tasty, succulent beef.

For almost a century Britain was known as 'stockyard to the world'. Today those once-great breeds are hard to find, even in their own native land. And the country that once set the standard for beef is no longer able to sell its own cattle.

The great merit of the traditional breeds was their efficiency in converting grass to beef. This is the job they were bred to do. Most were early maturing, which meant they 'finished' quickly with a good covering of fat. But it was a healthy kind of fat – rich in vitamins, minerals and polyunsaturated fats with their essential fatty acids.

In the 1970s, a number of events conspired to topple the native breeds from their elevated position as the main producers of the nation's beef. Animal fats were beginning to be stigmatized as the cause of heart disease. Suddenly the traditional breeds – whose very fats had given their meats such flavour – started to look suspect.

The fat theory of heart attacks is now largely discredited. Its proponents, writes James Le Fanu, glossed over the fact that the amount of fat in the diet predicted neither the cholesterol level nor the risk of heart disease in any single country.[15] The great cholesterol deception, as he calls it, was the result of the official endorsement of a false theory.

Nutritionist Sally Fallon believes that animal fats are not merely safe but a vital part of a healthy diet.[16] In addition to vitamins A and D, beef fat contains important fatty acids, she argues, including palmitoleic acid, an antimicrobial that protects against pathogens in the gut. It's also a good source of CLA, the powerful protector against cancer, but only if the beef animal has been grazing fresh pasture.

Back in the 1970s – when the animal fat/heart disease theory seemed incontestable – beef production went in precisely the wrong direction. The growing use of chemical fertilizers and pesticides was flooding the market with cheap, industrial cereal grains. Beef farmers spotted an economic advantage in using a larger animal – one that would be fast-growing but slower to mature than the native breeds. They could safely take such an animal to higher live weights without the risk of it becoming too fat. And best of all, it could be kept in a yard and fed on the new, cheaper cereals.

Turning their backs on the British breeds, farmers looked to continental Europe for their stock. Today, modern intensive beef production is dominated by breeds such as the Limousin, the Charolais, the Belgian Blue and the Simmental. They were imported to produce a large, lean carcass. The farmer would make money by growing them quickly on energy-rich diets, and the butcher would make money because they could be processed efficiently.

But the bold new era of beef production has done little for the eating quality of the product, or the health of consumers. Far from enhancing the real health benefits of beef, industrial production has done its best to obliterate them.

To find healthy beef today, it's necessary to search out meat from cattle raised on fertile, species-rich grassland. And they must have been on pasture for a substantial part of their lives, not just for a period in the middle of the fattening process. The longer an animal has run on grass the higher will be the level of omega-3 fats in the meat.

For the short period when cattle are housed for the winter, the diet should be made up chiefly of fibrous foods – hay or silage mainly, with some root crops and perhaps a small amount of barley. For safety, it's best to avoid anything that has been fed on soya, and for the very best tasting beef it's well worth seeking out one of the traditional native breeds.

7
The Fertile Soil

As a farming journalist, I worked for editors who liked referring to modern, chemical agriculture as 'scientific farming'. The implication was that traditional farming was in some way 'unscientific', or as in the old jibe, 'muck and magic'.

As I reiterate many times in this book, today's so-called scientific farming is based on an outdated science, the science of the mid-nineteenth century, and a blind adherence to it is squeezing the life from the soil. As I've explained, modern farmers, when they want to grow a crop, turn first to chemical fertilizers that supply the major plant nutrients – nitrogen, phosphorus and potassium – in a highly-soluble form. Crop plants are able to take them up quickly and produce a vigorous burst of growth, but the weakened tissue has to be sprayed with an array of pesticides to stop it succumbing to pests and diseases.

The chemical approach to feeding plants dates back to the early nineteenth century and to the work of a clever and charismatic German scientist, called Justus von Liebig. Since the time of Aristotle, philosophers had believed that plants were sustained by organic material gathered from the soil. Although this idea came under attack in the late-eighteenth century, it was Liebig who finally blew it out of the water.

In a paper to the British Association for the Advancement of Science, he put forward the theory that plants obtained their

For someone who once lost a modest fortune in the property market, Martin Lane seems a remarkably happy man. He went into property after a successful flying career in the RAF, and quickly made a pile. He then promptly lost it in the slump of the late 1980s.

Talking to him today, you almost feel he's glad. He runs a company called Field Science, which helps worried farmers restore the fertility of their worn-out soils. He's convinced he's part of a process that will cut the nation's health bills in half and give tens of thousands of people a fitter future. A spec like that is bound to provide a fair degree of job satisfaction.

I meet him one summer's afternoon in a gently rolling stretch of countryside. We've arranged to take a short walk. He has brought a trowel and I've brought my notebook.

The countryside he has chosen looks pleasant enough – mostly grass fields with plenty of hedges and trees. Seeing it from the road you'd think it was an unspoiled corner of pastoral England. Down at ground level things are far from unspoiled.

We climb the gate into a field with neat rows of young maize plants. Round here maize isn't grown for corn-on-the-cob. Dairy farmers harvest the whole plant and chop it up for silage to feed their cows, but the cows eating this particular crop are likely to go dangerously short of minerals.

Below the spindly-looking plants, the dry ground is covered with hard-baked clods of earth. Lane picks one up and examines it. The clod is about the size of a golf ball and just as hard. He tries in vain to push his thumbnail into it, but he makes no impression.

'Totally impenetrable,' he says. 'There's no plant root could break into that.' He tosses the piece away and begins scratching at the ground with his trowel. Beneath the clods is a thin layer of fine dust. Below that, what had once been soil is set solid as concrete. Here and there the light brown earth is mottled with reddish-brown. This is the subsoil showing through. At these points the valuable topsoil has all but eroded away.

'The structure's gone completely,' says Lane. 'Too many years of fertilizers, chemicals and heavy machines, and now it's finally given up. About all this soil can provide is a physical anchorage for plant roots. There'll be precious little nutrition in it.

'To make up for it the farmer will have to feed his cows an expensive mineral supplement. But supplements are never as effective, whether they're for livestock or for humans. Minerals are meant to be in our food. That's where they do most good.'

We walk across to a stile leading into the next field. This is pastureland with a good, thick growth of grass, but the grass is all the same. It is a monoculture of perennial ryegrass.

Once more Lane digs into the ground with his trowel. It's softer here than in the maize field. By working the trowel around he is able to bring up a sizeable lump of soil. It looks pretty solid – not at all the crumbly structure of a fertile soil, but at least it has a few grass roots running through it.

Lane's verdict is not good. 'The air spaces have mostly gone, which is a bad sign. There'll be a build-up of anaerobic conditions. That's the last thing you need for healthy plants. It's probably the result of high rates of nitrogen fertilizer. There's a fair chance the grass from this field won't have the minerals to keep cattle healthy.'

He spies something in the hedge bank – a bare patch of ground. Here is proof that the cows, which normally graze this pasture, aren't getting the nutrients they need.

In the bare earth of the bank, tongue marks are clearly visible. The animals have been licking bare soil from the hedge bank, the only place within reach where the earth hasn't been degraded. They needed minerals that were no longer supplied in the grass, and this was their only means of getting them. They were selecting their own mineral supplement.

Lane goes on: 'Our own diets have been depleted for exactly the same reasons. Take the trace element zinc. In the human body it's required in 300 different enzymes. Yet two-thirds of the population don't get enough of it.

'Then there's selenium. You can't be healthy without it. Yet the chemical industry is constantly urging farmers to put on ammonium sulphate fertilizer just because it's widely available as a chemical by-product, but there's growing evidence that it "locks up" selenium in the soil.

'A few years back the soil samples we took for our farmer customers almost always showed selenium to be present, even if it was only at a low level. Nowadays we're getting more and more samples with no measurable selenium.

'Is it any wonder that people are going down with degenerative diseases as soon as they hit middle age. It's the cumulative result of years of under-nutrition.'

This is a man not normally given to extravagant language. As a former RAF pilot he is trained in clear thinking. Yet he's convinced that a return to fertile soils and sound farming is needed to restore the health of both people and animals. With a possibility like that it's hard, he admits, not to get a little 'messianic' about the job.

We fight our way through a tall, straggling hedge into what is clearly another grass field, but that is where any similarity with the over-fertilized ryegrass pasture ends. This was a hay meadow, and though it is just yards away from the chemical grassland, it might be in another country.

Tall grass-heads of all shapes and sizes sway and tremble in the summer air. There must be a dozen or more different species. Scattered among them are a mass of brightly-coloured flowers – purple vetch, yellow buttercup and bird's-foot trefoil, tall red clover and scented meadowsweet.

I wonder what the neighbouring farmer must think as he glances across from his tractor cab while charging up and down with the fertilizer spreader. No doubt he shakes his head at this throwback to a backward and inefficient style of farming. Yet together these grasses and herbs are likely to provide all the minerals and nutrients cattle need without any requirement for expensive supplements.

Once more my companion digs into the ground with his trowel. Here it is soft and yielding. He pulls out a wedge of moist, crumbly soil. It is full of plant roots and in this one small sample there are two earthworms.

'If we kept all our soils like this we could grow anything,' he says. 'We'd use a lot less fertilizer and we'd hardly need any chemical sprays. And the food produced would be a great deal healthier for all of us.

'It's like they used to say. It's an old cliché, but the answer really does lie in the soil. Unfortunately, modern farming seems to have forgotten this.'

carbon, oxygen, hydrogen and nitrogen from the atmosphere, and the other elements they needed from the soil. These essential elements included iron, sulphur and phosphorus in the form of phosphates.

However, Liebig's theory was not perfect either. He was wrong about atmospheric hydrogen and – in the words of Colin Tudge, author of *So Shall We Reap* – 'spectacularly wrong' about nitrogen.[1] Liebig had proposed that ammonia produced by lightning in the upper atmosphere supplied all the nitrogen plants needed. After much argument he was forced to concede that this was not enough. Plants also needed some form of nitrogen at their roots.

Traditional agriculture depends on the recycling of nitrogen through the return of organic wastes to the soil. The other great providers of nitrogen are leguminous plants such as clover and beans, which form symbiotic relationships with soil bacteria of the genus rhizobium, capable of 'fixing' nitrogen from the atmosphere. By including legumes in their crop rotations, traditional farmers were able to boost the nitrogen fertility of their land. Otherwise the vast quantities of nitrogen present in the atmosphere were largely unavailable for crop production, except for a small amount converted to ammonia by lightning and carried into the soil with rainwater.

In spite of his error, Liebig produced a radical shift in thinking as he travelled up and down Britain lecturing to landowners and selling his own patent fertilizer – which didn't work. Through the power of his personality he demolished the idea that there was something special about living matter; that it contained some mysterious and indefinable 'life force'. Farming was simply a matter of calculating the amounts of essential elements removed in a crop at harvest time and replacing these in the soil with some form of soluble fertilizer.

Later in life, Liebig recanted his early dogmas. In notes written in 1843, he comes across as almost wretched:

I had sinned against the wisdom of our creator, and received just punishment for it. I wanted to improve his handiwork, and in my blindness, I believed that in his wonderful chain of laws, which ties life to the surface of the earth and always keeps it rejuvenated, there might be a link missing that had to be replaced by me – this weak powerless nothing.

Whatever his own misgivings, his philosophy became rooted in a Britain gripped by the possibilities of science and industrialism. Today's farming is built on the habit of applying the major plant nutrients – nitrogen, phosphorus and potassium – in the form of chemical salts. It has become known as the NPK philosophy (after the three letters symbolizing these elements), and the chemical industry – which benefits handsomely from it – has succeeded in spreading it around the world.

Around the world traditional farming – based on recycled animal and vegetable wastes – has been swept aside before the relentless advance of chemical agriculture. Chemical farming is leading the world to a precipice. It is bound to fail because it has ignored the one element that can ensure human health – the life of the soil.

Liebig and his modern disciples were wrong in assuming that

the flooding of crop roots with soluble salts would lead to healthy plant growth. Fertile soils produce healthy growth. And soils don't become fertile just because they contain high levels of organic matter and available minerals. To promote healthy growth they also need large populations of microbes and other soil organisms – an underground army, which is constantly breaking down and rebuilding nutrients from plant and animal wastes; and in the process making minerals available to plants. About 5 per cent of soil is composed of organic matter – the wastes and decomposed residues of plants and animals, together with the billions of organisms that live in the air spaces between mineral particles.

It is the actions of this living community that enable plants to grow. They supply plants with the nutrients they need, provide them with water and protect them against toxins and disease. Without the activity of soil organisms – from microscopic bacteria to earthworms – life on the planet would quickly grind to a halt. Chemical farming subjects these living communities to a non-stop toxic barrage, wiping out whole species and disrupting the intricate, below-ground network that keeps plants healthy.

With their natural support systems severely weakened, crop plants become more dependent on pesticides to keep them growing – which is great news for the chemical industry. Many agricultural soils are now so damaged by chemical fertilizers and pesticides that they need ever greater amounts to produce any crop at all. They've been turned into agrochemical junkies, wholly dependent on the local chemical supplier for the next fix.

Sometimes when you kick over a clod of earth, it's hard to grasp the complexity of it. We often call it dirt. Unlike 'land', with its real estate connotations, we attach little value to soil, but it keeps us fed and would – if only we looked after it better – take care of our health.

Just a teaspoonful of healthy soil contains over five billion living organisms, representing 10,000 or so different species. Most are anonymous, like the crowds in a city street. The world a few inches beneath our feet is no better known than the life of deep oceans.

What is known is that bacteria are likely to be the most numerous group in the teaspoon of fertile soil. There will be two to three billion of them. In size and activity they'll range from the rhizobia – the family which 'fixes' atmospheric nitrogen in special nodules in plant roots – to the threadlike actinomycetes that appear more like fungi.

Bacteria get a bad press in our society, mainly because there are dozens of companies trying to sell us products to wipe them out. But of the billions of bacteria in the soil the vast majority are beneficial. They are involved in almost all metabolic processes that go on below ground. Malign species only cause trouble when the soil has been so badly mismanaged that its normal life breaks down. That's their job – to clear up the mess.

Next in complexity come the protozoa – there are likely to be around 50,000 of them in that teaspoon of healthy soil. These single-cell animals feed mostly on bacteria from which they differ in having at least one well-defined cell nucleus. They're classed according to the way they travel through water – amoebae get about by the flowing movement of their protoplasm, ciliates by the wave motions of their hair-like cilia, and flagellates by the rapid flexing of their whip-like flagella.

Another abundant group are the soil fungi, which may be single-cell yeasts or the more complex multi-cellular moulds. These filamentous fungi are made up of long, branching chains of cells known as hyphae, which may be interwoven to form mycelia, the thin, white strands sometimes visible to the naked eye in leaf litter. Filamentous fungi break down most types of organic material, from tree bark to decaying animal remains. Some species form symbiotic relationships with plants roots, supplying the plant with some of the essential elements it needs in exchange for energy-rich secretions from the root.

Nematodes also play a key role in the below-ground drama. This group is essentially made up of worms – roundworms, threadworms and eelworms. Originally water dwellers, some forms migrated to land and became adapted to living in the pores and films of water between soil particles. Farmers see nematodes as the enemy, mainly because they include crop pests such as the potato cyst eelworm. But in well-managed soils, nematodes aid crop production by helping to recycle nutrients and by keeping root-eating species like the potato eelworm in check.

Of the more visible players in the drama, earthworms are the stars. Charles Darwin wrote his final book on the subject of earthworms.[2] He showed that the collapse and partial burial of many of the great monumental stones at Stonehenge had been the result of earthworm activity over many centuries.

Britain has twenty-five species, of which ten are common. An earthworm can live for up to five years, ingesting many times its own weight of soil each day. In doing so it creates a network of pores, which improve drainage and soil aeration. Along the walls it secretes calcium-rich mucus, and from time to time it expels casts containing a range of plant nutrients. Plant roots snake their way through these underground channels, making good use of the nutrient-rich deposits so conveniently left for them.

If earthworms are the stars of the larger soil animals, there are many others playing supporting roles. Among them are soil arthropods, including mites, springtails and beetles. This group is important in breaking up organic wastes and starting off the process of nutrient recycling. A good example is the dung beetle, which stores balls of nutrient-rich animal dung in shallow, underground channels.

In Darwinian terms, these myriad life forms are locked in an unending struggle for survival and genetic immortality. Yet the outcome is seldom – as in human economic systems – the emergence of a few dominant players. A sudden catastrophic change in conditions may lead to a collapse in some species, but the natural response of the soil community is to stabilize the situation and restore diversity.

For all its savage competition, the soil acts almost as a single organism spread across the land surface of the planet. Within it the ceaseless building up and breaking down of living matter accumulates minerals and locks them in the system so they are not leached away in the groundwater. And it creates humus, the group of long-chain carbon compounds, which links with clay particles to form a fine, crumb structure. In short, it maintains the perfect conditions for terrestrial life.

Down through the ages – with no knowledge of science – farmers have striven to build up the life of their soils. The more active the life of the soil the greater the store of nutrients for crop growth. In a fertile pasture producing meat or milk, there'll be at least twice the weight of 'stock' below ground than there is grazing on the surface vegetation.

In the ancient wisdom of the fields, farmers have always known this. The return of animal and plant wastes as manure and compost was aimed at stimulating the life of the soil. Bacteria and soil fungi need a constant flow of organic material to work on or their numbers will quickly fall. When this happens, nutrients are lost from the system. In extreme cases the structure breaks down and the soil dies.

Most of the mechanisms through which soil organisms nurture crop plants remain shrouded in mystery, but at Oregon State University, microbiologist Professor Elaine Ingham has started to provide answers.[3] Pared down to its essentials fertility depends on the balance between decomposers – organisms such as bacteria, fungi and certain arthropods that break down soil organic matter – and their predators.

The decomposers are responsible for holding nutrients in the topsoil so they're not washed away in the groundwater. As they get to work on organic matter in the soil, the nutrients the decomposers release are incorporated into their body tissue. Bacteria and fungi together account for a large proportion of the nitrogen, phosphorus, sulphur and other minerals safely secured in the topsoil.

For these minerals to become available to plants once more they must first be freed back into the soil through the process of mineralization. This is where the predators come in. They include groups such as protozoa, nematodes, small arthropods and earthworms, which feed on the bacteria and fungi. In doing so they release much of the nitrogen and other minerals so that these are available to plants.

Together protozoa and nematodes regulate the process of

mineralization. But their numbers in turn are controlled by a higher order of predators such as millipedes, centipedes, beetles, spiders and small mammals. It's this constant mêlée of life forms – from the simplest to the advanced – that is the foundation of fertility, the provider of plenty and the guarantor of health. Elaine Ingham calls it the soil food web. The greater its complexity – the more momentous the underground struggle between predator and prey – the more the earth will produce.

But the farming methods of industrial countries seem designed to wreck this ordered complexity. Chemical fertilizers, pesticides, soil fungicides and fumigants (which sterilize the soil) – the whole arsenal used by industrial farmers in their battle with nature – all kill bacteria and fungi. Overwhelmingly, it's the beneficial species that are hit hardest. That's when disease organisms seize the opportunity to strike at crops.

It's a similar story to the overuse of antibiotics. When antibiotics were first introduced they seemed to offer a miracle cure for some of the world's worst disease scourges. As they were used more widely drug-resistant organisms began to appear. At the same time, beneficial bugs were knocked out by the indiscriminate new products, leaving the field clear for more malign organisms.

In the same way, when chemical fertilizers or pesticides take out bacteria and fungi in the soil, a host of dependent organisms vanish along with them. Predators are knocked out with prey species. Soon the soil ecosystem starts to break down. The normal checks and balances no longer work and disease-causing species move into the vacant space.

The best way to take care of healthy soils is to heap on organic materials – straw and crop residues, manures and composts. A soil that's fertile and productive doesn't need chemical fertilizers or pesticides.

A Cornell University study of America's longest-running investigation into organic farming showed that getting rid of pesticide sprays and chemical fertilizers leads to more biological activity in the soil, and ultimately to more food at lower cost.[4]

Led by David Pimental, the study looked at a twenty-two-year-long trial at the Rodale Institute in Pennsylvania. In it chemical farming of corn and soya beans was compared with an organic rotation where no chemicals were used.

The research team compared the activity of soil fungi on the two systems as well as a number of other aspects, including crop yields, energy efficiency, costs and the level of organic matter. The organic system produced yields that were as high as those of the chemical system, but they achieved it with 30 per cent less energy, less water and no pesticides. Crop yields on the organic system were particularly high in drought years. This was because wind and water erosion degraded the soil on the chemical system. On the organic soil, by contrast, the level of organic matter steadily rose along with moisture levels and the activity of soil micro-organisms.

Though they wouldn't have understood the science, farmers down the ages fed soil organisms with organic material, in effect taking care of the soil ecosystem and allowing the soil to provide their crops.

Former farmer John Reeves learned the hard way that soil organisms are vital to the health of plants and animals. In the early 1980s, he gave up his Devon farm and set off with his wife Kate and three children, Charlotte, William and Ben, to begin a new life sheep-farming in western Canada. The farm they bought on Vancouver Island had been cleared from forest over the previous thirty years. The climate was benign – not unlike that of eastern England – and the native forest vegetation grew thick and lush. The family had every reason to expect a bright and rewarding future. Instead, the next few years turned into nightmare.

Their lambs were born stunted and sickly. They failed to thrive and fattening them for the market proved almost impossible. Next there was a near epidemic of broken legs among the flock. That's when Reeves began to suspect a mineral imbalance.

There was a crop of other ailments. Some lambs developed white muscle disease, a form of dystrophy in which the legs become stiff and swollen. It is corrected with an injection of selenium. Other lambs developed sway-back, a type of paralysis caused by the poor development of myelin, the insulating material that surrounds the central nervous system (see page 59). It's preventable so long as the ewe obtains adequate levels of copper in the diet.

Each year there would be several cases of thiamine – vitamin B_1 – deficiency. Animals would drop on their sides, their heads pressed back and their front legs pedalling the air. By now Reeves had become convinced that mineral imbalances lay at the heart of his problems. He started feeding his animals special supplements to restore the missing nutrients. At last the flock became healthy again, but the losses had cost the family most of their savings. They were forced to sell up and return to Britain.

Chastened by the experience Reeves spent the next twenty years carrying out his own research on soil minerals, and the way they're taken up by crops. He's now convinced of the vital role played by one particular group of soil organisms – mycorrhiza. Without them plants can't take up all the minerals they need so the animals – and people eating them – are more likely to become sick. But it's a group of organisms that industrial agriculture has done its best to obliterate.

The organisms identified as vital by John Reeves are known collectively as mycorrhiza. They're thread-like fungi that form intimate links with plant roots, actually penetrating the cells of the root cortex. It's a mutually beneficial arrangement known in biology as symbiosis. The plant supplies the fungus with carbohydrates and amino acids in its sap. In return the fungus supplies the plant with minerals, helps it to resist drought and protects it against soil-borne diseases and harmful nematodes.

In effect, mycorrhiza form an extension of the plant's root

system. There are thought to be seven groups of the fungus, most of which are specialized for particular plant families. The largest group is the vesicular-arbuscular mycorrhizae (VAM), so called because they form little sac-like structures – or arbuscules – inside the root cells. These increase the surface area across which the plant can trade nutrients for minerals. The VAM can increase the absorbing surface of the plant's root hairs by up to one hundred thousand times. And they can enhance the uptake of soil nutrients such as phosphorus, zinc, copper and magnesium by up to sixty times. That's why these little-known organisms are so essential to human health.

Mycorrhiza are thought to have evolved more than 300 million years ago, in evolutionary terms not long after the appearance of land plants. They evolved to form symbiotic links with the roots of most plant species.

Biologists have known about them for a century. Because of the power of the chemical industry they've been largely ignored. But thanks to the conviction and dogged determination of an amateur scientist, the human cost of that neglect is becoming clear.

I tracked down John Reeves in a tucked-away cottage on the edge of a small community in the Forest of Dean in Gloucestershire. Since he returned from Canada he has carried out dozens of experiments on plant minerals. His aim was to find out how the presence or absence of mycorrhiza in the soil affects the mineral content of the crops it grows. He admits to being sceptical at the start. The idea that a soil fungus could have a significant influence on the nutritional quality – as well as the yield – of a crop seemed fanciful.

He's sceptical no longer. Today he's convinced we'll never again eat healthy foods until we return to a system of farming that protects these valuable organisms. And that means getting rid of most of our chemical fertilizers and sprays.

He carried out his experiments on a number of different soils, though many were done on his own land, a magnesium limestone soil to the south of the Forest of Dean. He enlisted the help of a university chemist to carry out the mineral analyses on his plant samples. A sympathetic scientist at

Rothamsted experimental station in Hertfordshire supplied the inoculum of mycorrhiza.

Reeves devised his own 'mineral score' to represent the overall content of fourteen essential trace elements, including boron, cobalt, copper, iron, magnesium, zinc and selenium. He included in his trials a range of everyday vegetables – carrots, peas, onions, parsnips, potatoes and broad beans.

When the vegetables were grown on cultivated soils without chemical fertilizers their mineral scores were satisfactory, though not high. But when they were grown on soils that had been treated with chemical fertilizer – phosphate – they contained up to a quarter fewer minerals.

Inoculating soils with mycorrhiza had the opposite effect – the mineral scores soared. Comparing the two treatments, vegetables grown on soils with healthy populations of mycorrhiza contained up to two-thirds more minerals than those from soils fertilized by chemicals.

Reeves also looked at a number of farm crops, including wheat and pasture grass. As with vegetables, both the physical act of cultivating the soil – and the application of chemical fertilizers – destroyed mycorrhiza and depleted growing crops of minerals.

With wheat he found that soil cultivation reduced the mineral content of grain by 25 per cent. Putting on chemical fertilizer reduced mineral levels still further, but when the cultivated soil was inoculated with mycorrhiza it again grew wheat containing the full complement of minerals.

Reeves made similar observations of pasture grasses. Grass leaves taken from long-established pasture contained high levels of essential trace elements, but when soils were sown back to grassland after five years of cultivation for crops, the resulting grass showed far lower levels of minerals. Selenium was reduced to almost half, boron and molybdenum by around 40 per cent, cobalt and copper by 30 per cent, and manganese and nickel by 20 per cent or more.[5]

Reeves believes his results show why there is so much ill health in western societies. They have relied on chemical fertilizers to grow most of their food. Yet those same chemicals

– particularly phosphates – destroy the natural system for growing healthy, nutrient-filled crops.

And if that weren't enough, most farmers rely on fungicide sprays to deal with diseases on their crops. The irony is that these chemicals are also likely to be killing the very soil fungi that could prevent their crops becoming diseased in the first place.

Looking back, Reeves attributes the failure of his sheep-farming venture to the absence of the *right species* of mycorrhiza on his land. It had been newly reclaimed from the forest so the fungal species present would have been those adapted to forest trees. Even if they survived they'd have been unable to establish a symbiotic association with grass roots. This is why the pastures were depleted in minerals and the animals became sick.

All this was known by farmers a century-and-a-half ago. In 1850, James Caird – a leading farming commentator – was commissioned by *The Times* to undertake a survey of English agriculture. In his report from Hertfordshire he describes a system for 'inoculating' new grassland so it will quickly become productive. Though the farmer he visited would not have understood the science, the technique ensured that the new pasture contained the right types of mycorrhiza for healthy and nutritious grass.

A small plough is passed along an old pasture, from which it throws out about three inches of turf and leaves a little more, returning again with another strip of turf, of the same breadth, until the requisite quantity is obtained. A corn drill is then passed over the ground to be inoculated, the coulters of which mark it off in rows at eight inches apart. The sod is then cut into little pieces and laid down in the rows, each piece about four inches apart, by men who then tread it into the ground. This must be done in damp weather in September or October. In spring the ground is rolled and a little Dutch clover is sown, after which the whole is allowed to seed itself, and stock is put on in autumn. By this process a fine pasture is rapidly formed.[6]

As mentioned earlier, today the essential role of mycorrhiza in maintaining the nutrient content of crops has been forgotten. According to Reeves, modern farming methods are fast destroying soil organisms that have supported plant life for millions of years. He explains: 'There's no need for pesticides or chemical fertilizers. By inoculating soils with mycorrhiza we could easily restore the natural systems that keep plants healthy and adequately supplied with minerals. Our crops would be protected against disease, and the foods they produced would be rich in nutrients.

'It's not credible that plants, animals and humans could have evolved with the requirement for higher levels of minerals than were provided by nature, but until we restore these natural systems we can't rely on the food supply to deliver them.'

Reeves wants to see food producers introduce quality controls for their products that take account of nutrient content as well as cosmetic appearance. In the meantime, he believes, consumers will have to rely on mineral supplements to make up the shortfall in everyday foods.

The chemist who analysed the mineral content of plants in Reeves's investigation was by Neil Ward, of Surrey University's School of Biomedical Molecular Science. Ward, too, thinks the re-introduction of mycorrhiza in agriculture would do much to enhance the nutrient status of foods.

A New Zealander, he grew up in a farming community where many of his relatives still farm. As a result of the UK trial, he suggested that an uncle farming in an arid region of New Zealand try using mycorrhiza to improve the pastures.

The advice proved very sound. Inoculation of the soil with the beneficial fungi resulted in an immediate improvement, Ward reports, with the turf growing thicker and lusher.

He'd like to see mycorrhiza sold in garden centres throughout Britain, though he has no great hopes that mainstream agriculture will embrace the technique. The chemical industry has too much to lose. With his colleague John Reeves, he has made the findings available to Defra, the Department for the Environment, Food and Rural Affairs. So far there has been no government commitment to research funding.

Ward is currently involved in research on the use of mycor-rhiza to establish grasslands in arid regions of several South American countries. While there's plenty of backing for the development of genetically-modified crops in such areas, there's less interest in mycorrhiza, the natural way of protect-ing plants in unfavourable climatic conditions.

In Scotland, I called to see another amateur farming sleuth who's convinced chemical farming damages our food. Former farmer Tom Stockdale once worked for the fertilizer company ICI. Now he thinks the high-nitrogen fertilizers sold by che-mical companies have harmed many UK soils. As a result they've been the cause of ill health among both human and animal populations.

He has good grounds for his claim. During his time as a farmer he became gravely ill as a result of a mineral imbal ance. The crisis spurred him to carry out a detailed study of soils and the way they're managed. Today he's more than ever convinced that the wide-scale use of high-nitrogen ferti-lizers is neither safe nor sustainable. And he fears the world's much-vaunted 'green revolution' – with its dependence on fertilizer nitrogen – is doomed to fail.

Stockdale is now retired, though his interest in soils and their effects on health remains undimmed. I met him in his solid, stone-built house on the outskirts of Dumfries. The day I called, the dining table was covered with technical books and papers, so we chatted in the sun-filled conservatory.

The son of a Cambridge chemistry don, he has had a life-long passion for farming. With his Cambridge agriculture diploma, he joined ICI in the late 1950s. He recalls with a wry smile that the day he started with the company was April Fools' Day.

'I was interested in the science of farming, but ICI was mainly interested in selling fertilizer. So it was pretty obvious we weren't going to be together for long.

'Up until that time most fertilizers were impure, which was an advantage in that it meant they contained trace elements.

For example, most farmers used basic slag, a by-product of the steel industry containing a lot of minerals. But ICI were just introducing their new, high-nitrogen fertilizers, so pure they contained no trace elements.

'The company was pushing them hard. Selling fertilizers wasn't a job I relished, so we decided – as a family – to go farming.'

Tom and his wife Margaret took the tenancy of a small hill farm in Scotland. There he started applying all 'the wonderful new methods' he'd learned at ICI, especially the use of high-nitrogen fertilizer. It soon became apparent something was going badly wrong.

His barley crops germinated well, then quickly began losing ground. The plants were stunted and the leaves turned purple. The plant roots were short and jagged – 'fanged' is how he describes them. Eventually the plants became so frail and light that they seemed about to blow away.

At the same time, the black coats of his Aberdeen Angus cattle started turning a dirty brown colour. Many of them 'scoured' – the cattle equivalent of getting diarrhoea. Slowly their grazing fields were taken over by moss.

A farm advisor he'd called in to help criticised him for failing to control the weeds in his crops, although he'd already sprayed them many times. After each dose of herbicide the weeds seemed to come back stronger than ever, even though the crops had failed. In desperation he resorted to even stronger – and more expensive – weedkillers, all to no avail.

It wasn't just the livestock that were ailing. Soon Stockdale himself became ill. On two occasions he was poisoned by the element molybdenum after it had found its way into the farm's private water supply.

When soils become anaerobic – lacking in oxygen – and lose their structure, the living processes that normally regulate the release of minerals break down. So potentially toxic elements such as molybdenum appear in ionic form in the soil water to act as rogue poisons.

After a while Stockdale began to feel awful. He recalled, 'It creeps up on you gradually. You don't really notice it at first. Then suddenly you're lacking in energy and having to drag yourself around. I got to the point that I didn't even dare glance in the mirror because I looked so awful.

'Not long after, we began eating wholemeal bread made from locally-grown flour. One by one we all became ill again. The doctor said it was due to infection with the *E. coli* bacterium. But I was convinced I'd developed type-two diabetes plus coeliac disease, where you're unable to digest fat. The symptoms are awful.

'Eventually we gave up the wholemeal bread and started to feel a bit better. By then we were talking to soil mineral specialists about the cause of the sickness in our cattle and crops. One of them said my own symptoms sounded like a selenium deficiency. So we all started taking selenium tablets. And very quickly all the symptoms disappeared.'

Since the health crisis Stockdale has spent many years studying the role of selenium in the metabolism of plants and animals, and the way chemical fertilizers disrupt natural processes. The findings have confirmed his belief that today's heavy use of high-nitrogen fertilizers is leading Britain – and other countries – to a health disaster.

When high-nitrogen fertilizers were introduced back in the 1960s they were tested mainly on the alkaline soils of southern and eastern England. On the basis of these findings, the fertilizer companies introduced recommendations for their use across the country. However, most UK soils are not alkaline but acid. They're on the igneous and metamorphic rocks that make up the bulk of the country. In these areas, high-nitrogen fertilizers damage soil structure and produce crops that are depleted of minerals.

It's a deficiency of selenium that worries Tom Stockdale most. Since his own illness he has become an expert on the physiological affects. With insufficient selenium the body is unable to activate the thyroid hormone thyroxine, he says. The body is starved of energy and any of a number of vital functions is likely to break down.

A marginal deficiency of selenium over many years can lead to coronary heart disease, he says, while those severely affected can suffer conditions such as obesity, depression and late-onset diabetes.[7] Some of these conditions can induce stress leading to panic attacks or outbreaks of irrational anger.

Chemical farming is portrayed as a great triumph of western technology because it produces mountains of grain and tanker-loads of milk. But it's hardly a triumph to ruin the nation's health. And who can take pride in a system that destroys the Earth's most precious asset – its soil?

8
In Praise of Yellow Butter

Today, milk and dairy products are demonized by diet propagandists. This is because a large proportion of their fats are in the form of saturated fats, and these are believed to be unhealthy. The idea originates from the theory developed in the 1950s and 60s – that animal fats and cholesterol in foods raise blood cholesterol, which then builds up in the arteries to cause heart disease. The theory has now been largely debunked.[1] Experimental evidence finally refuting it emerged in the early 1980s.[2]

Far from being harmful, saturated fats play an important role in human nutrition. They enhance the immune system, protect against pathogens, provide energy to the heart and are essential to the function of the kidneys and lungs.[3] Despite this, many still believe saturated fats to be bad.

As if this weren't enough, a growing number of people appear to be intolerant of milk. Medical journals have run a string of articles on milk allergies in babies and young children. What the authors don't reveal is that almost all these allergies are to pasteurized milk.

A century ago a diet of unpasteurized, whole milk was widely recommended as the cure to a range of conditions, including diabetes, gastric ulcers, obesity and kidney disease. In the United States, a doctor called Charles Sanford Porter published *Milk Diet as a Remedy for Chronic Disease*, a book

On the edge of the Bernese Oberland in the Swiss Alps lies a hidden valley accessible through a long rail tunnel. Before the coming of the railway in about 1910, the only way to reach the Loetschental was on foot via a high mountain pass. The people living in the string of small villages spread along the valley floor subsisted entirely on the foods they could grow in their remote mountain world.

Hung on a wall of the tiny museum at Kippel, there's a group photograph of children at the village school in about 1900. Posing unsmiling in their worn, hand-me-down clothes, they're clearly from a community well used to poverty. Yet without exception the children – whose ages range from about six to fourteen – look remarkably healthy.

None are obese. Nor are they thin and gaunt. Their faces are wide and well-fleshed in contrast to the pinched and drawn features seen in many contemporary photographs from schools in Britain's industrial cities. These Swiss youngsters were obviously well-nourished.

Close to the village museum stands a small church with an immaculately-kept burial ground. This is likely to have been the last resting place of at least some of the children in the picture. The dates on the headstones show that many incumbents were born in the latter years of the nineteenth century. Of these most survived into their seventies and eighties. A few lived into their nineties and one had survived to be over one hundred.

The children in the school photograph appear to have lived long and healthy lives, though few will have enjoyed the benefits of modern medicine. What kept them fit and active was their food. In their early years, at least, the bulk of their diet was made up chiefly of local dairy products, supplemented with a little meat plus the fruits and vegetables they had grown on their village plots. Today dairy products, with their heavy loading of saturated fats, are viewed with suspicion. In the current medical orthodoxy, they're foods to be taken in moderation. Yet these mountain people ate large amounts of them and lived long and active lives. But the butter and cheese produced in this isolated Alpine valley were very different from those most of us eat today.

They were from the milk of cows grazing flower-strewn Alpine pastures, meaning they contained many vitamins and minerals, far more than milk today. Modern milk is from cows bred to produce huge quantities, on feeds very different from the fresh grass evolution had adapted them for.

that ran to eleven editions. In it he wrote: 'A good food is a good remedy, and, as disease is only a disturbance of the mechanism of nutrition, it is only natural that the use of milk in ill health should be almost as old as its use as a food in health.'[4]

Porter insisted that the milk must be unpasteurized. 'What is required is good, clean milk as it comes from the cow, without the removal or addition of any substance whatsoever. Boiled, sterilized or pasteurized milk – or milk artificially preserved in any way – cannot be used for this treatment. Pasteurizing milk renders it unsuitable for human use.'

There's a sound basis for Porter's argument. Pasteurization destroys milk enzymes, which would otherwise help the body assimilate nutrients, including calcium.[5] It also destroys the lactic-acid-producing bacteria which protect against pathogens. It destroys vitamins and makes many of milk's most valuable trace elements less available.

In 1929, Dr J.R. Crewe of the Mayo Foundation in Rochester, Minnesota, published an article on the benefits of milk in the *Certified Milk Magazine*.[6] In it he claimed to have used unpasteurized milk to improve a variety of health conditions, including obesity, heart disease, diabetes, prostrate enlargement, tuberculosis and high blood pressure.

The drinking of unpasteurized milk is not to be recommended where there is any risk of the herd being infected with bovine TB, as is sadly the case in some regions of Britain. But modern science has confirmed the health benefits of milk and dairy foods that are produced in the traditional way from the milk of cows grazing on fertile, fast-growing pastures (see below).

Cows are adapted to eating grass. It is their natural food. Evolution has equipped them with a large fermentation chamber – the rumen – in which fibrous materials, low in energy, are broken down by resident micro-organisms. This is, after all, why human beings domesticated them in the first place. Ruminants have the capacity to convert inedible roughages into food.

In Europe, cows were traditionally calved in spring. So the peak demand for milk came at the time when the growth of fresh green grass was at its most vigorous. As Weston Price discovered in Switzerland in the 1930s (see Chapter 2), many rural peoples placed a special value on the deep yellow butter made from the milk of cows feeding on this early spring grass. They knew intuitively that its life-enhancing qualities were especially beneficial to children and expectant mothers.

Milk from cows feeding on young fresh grass contains high levels of the fat-soluble vitamins A, D, K and E. So butter made from this milk is a rich source. Vitamin A is more easily absorbed from butter than from other foods.

Vitamins A and E are powerful antioxidants. They protect the body against damaging pollutants and free radicals, so acting as anti-cancer agents.

Vitamin D – like vitamin A – is needed for calcium and phosphorus absorption. It is essential for strong bones and teeth, and for normal growth. Vitamin K is a key factor in blood clotting. Like the other fat-soluble vitamins, it also plays a role in bone formation.

Milk from grass-fed cows contains high levels of essential fatty acids, particularly omega-3 fatty acid and the restructured linoleic acid known as conjugated linoleic acid (CLA), with its strong anti-cancer properties. Even small amounts of milk and cheese from pasture-fed cows has been linked to a significant fall in the cancer risk. One researcher estimated that eating one serving daily of grass-fed meat, plus one ounce of cheese and one glass of whole milk from a grass-fed cow could significantly reduce the risk of cancer.[7]

CLA is produced in large amounts by cows eating fresh, green grass.[8] But when cows are fed on small amounts of grain – or even on grass that has been cut and conserved in the form of silage – its level in milk falls away dramatically.[9] There's even evidence that old pastures containing plants like plantain, self-heal, rough hawk bit, red clover and bird's-foot trefoil produced milk with higher CLA levels than all-grass pastures.[10]

Organically produced milk is known to be richer in nutrients than conventional milk because, under European law, organic dairy farmers are required to feed a high proportion of home-grown forage feeds to their cattle. In practice this means cows spend a lot of time grazing on grass and clover pastures. As a result, organic milk has been found to be 50 per cent higher in vitamin E, 75 per cent higher in beta-carotene (converted in the body to vitamin A) and two to three times higher in the antioxidants lutein and zeaxanthine.[11]

Research at the University of Aberdeen showed that levels of omega-3 fats were, on average, 30 per cent higher in organic milk than in non-organic milk.[12] But the differences were far higher in the summer months when the organically farmed cows had greater access to fresh grass and clover-rich pastures.

Without the benefit of modern scientific knowledge, the traditional dairy farmers of Europe knew their summer pastures delivered the healthiest and most nutritious dairy foods. It's a belief that persisted into the mid-twentieth century. A Dairy Council ad of the time showed three young boys sharing a glass of milk. The caption read: 'You'll feel a lot better if you drink more milk.'

Today's dairy advertising still targets young people. On its stand at the 2004 Dairy Event – the national show for UK dairy farmers – the Milk Development Council displayed life-sized cutouts of two smiling teenage girls. Surveys had shown they were the group most likely to be short of calcium in their diet. In response, the industry's 'Three a day' campaign warned that low-calcium diets could lead to osteoporosis in later life. Three portions of milk, yogurt or cheese every day were a simple way to meet calcium requirements, said the ad. Among other benefits, milk and dairy products were claimed to give protection against colon and breast cancer, a benefit thought to be linked to their calcium and vitamin D content.[13]

What the ads don't tell you is that damaging changes in the way milk is produced have depleted it of the very vitamins the body needs to take up calcium in the diet. So that far from enhancing its natural, cancer-fighting properties, the changes have blunted them.

In a little over a generation, dairy farming has been transformed from a natural process into an industrial operation. In that time the health benefits of milk have been systematically eroded, and the role of the dairy cow has changed from one of generous companion to abused and over-exploited slave.

In the 1960s, the average yield of a British dairy cow was a little over 3,500 litres a year. Today the average is almost double this, with some high-production herds notching up 10,000 litres or more. The cow is able to transfer only a fixed amount of vitamins to her milk. The greater her milk volume, the more dilute its vitamin content, particularly for vitamin E and beta-carotene, a precursor of vitamin A. The 'unimproved' cows may have put less milk in the tank at the end of every day, but while they were grazing fresh pasture it was milk packed with nutrients.

The modern Holstein super-cow is little more than a walking milk generator. To achieve these levels of output, the cattle breeders have selected from animals with over-active pituitary glands. The pituitary not only secretes hormones that stimulate the production of milk, it also produces growth hormones. These inevitably turn up in the milk. High levels of pituitary hormones have been linked to the formation of tumours.[14]

The development of what nutritionist Sally Fallon calls the 'freak pituitary cow' has led to dramatic changes in the way herds are fed. Grass – the natural food of ruminants – is unable to provide the energy-rich and protein-dense rations these high-performance animals need in their genetically-programmed drive to produce vast quantities of milk. Unless they are fed nutrients in concentrated form they will break down their own body tissue to the point of collapse.

No longer can they be left to graze pasture alone for a large part of the year. Grass must now be supplemented with a range of industrial feeds, many of which spoil the nutritional value of the milk.

Cereals such as wheat, maize and barley are among the starchy foods chosen to boost energy levels in the diet of high-yielding cows. These industrial grains are cheap and plentiful. But there are other, equally damaging foods on offer – potato waste; bread discarded by the factory bakers; breakfast cereals that for one reason or another have been rejected for the human food chain.

These energy-rich foods have to be 'balanced' with feeds supplying concentrated forms of protein. This is why dairy farmers embarked on the disastrous practice of feeding meat-and-bone meal to their cows – a move that may have caused the spread of 'mad cow disease' and its human equivalent. Had dairy farmers not chosen to base their production on abnormal cows they wouldn't have needed to resort to abnormal diets to sustain their excessive output.

Today farmers rely heavily on soya bean meal to supply protein in concentrated form. Unfortunately most soya – like cereals – is grown with heavy inputs of pesticide and chemical fertilizer. Other widely-used protein feeds include groundnut meal, rapeseed meal and cottonseed meal.

On today's factory farms, grazed grass – the cow's natural food – produces less than one-sixth of the milk that goes into the food chain. The rest is produced from other feed materials. That's why our dairy foods no longer have the health-giving properties of those from that remote Swiss valley (see page 124).

The healthy omega-3 fats of grass-fed milk are largely eliminated on these industrial rations. Instead the milk fat is almost entirely made up of saturated fats. These high-octane rations also depress the levels of CLA in milk, so reducing its protective effects against cancer. Fat-soluble vitamins are re-duced; so are the antioxidants lutein and zeaxanthine.

This finding explains why milk produced by traditional methods was so widely regarded as a healthy food. As pointed out earlier, under the rules of organic production, cows eat large amounts of fresh grass and clover, just as they did on the Swiss mountainside.

Taking ruminants off grass is as damaging for dairy cows as it is for beef cattle. Too much starchy food in the diet increases the acidity of the cow's rumen, particularly when it's fed in large amounts. The rumen microbes respond by producing excess lactic acid, some of which is absorbed into the blood-stream where it disrupts the animal's normal metabolism.

Toxins, too, are released into the bloodstream. These are produced by the decay of micro-organisms killed in the over-acid conditions. Other pathogenic microbes seize the oppor-tunity and multiply. This is why high-yielding cows are beset by ill health.

There are dangers for consumers, too. In the highly-acid intestinal conditions of cows fed mainly on grain, the bacteria that thrive include the acid-resistant pathogens most harmful to human beings. Among the most dangerous is the *E. coli* strain 0157. It takes as few as ten organisms to cause illness, even death in humans. Their numbers in cattle fed inside on grain and silage are far higher than in cattle fed mainly on grass and hay.[15]

Disease is endemic in modern intensive dairy units. As much as 40 per cent of the national herd suffers from some form of mastitis or udder infection. A Bristol University survey put the average incidence of clinical mastitis in Britain's dairy cows at almost 70 per cent.[16] This means they are secreting pus cells into the milk, which ends up in our 'healthy' yogurt or milk shake.

In a bid to limit the epidemic, farmers routinely squirt antibiotics up the teats of their cows during the 'dry' period – the short period between lactation cycles – but antibiotics deal with the symptoms, not with the cause of disease. Cows are too often ill because of the way they're managed.

Faulty feeding lies behind another modern affliction of dairy cows – lameness. Around a quarter of the national dairy herd suffers from lameness, commonly caused by a restriction in the blood supply to the feet. Toxins and histamines in the blood –

the result of over-acidic conditions in the rumen – permanently damage the blood vessels supplying the tissues of the foot. As a result, the feet of many modern dairy cows are susceptible to damage and infection.

As if this weren't enough, the stresses on these high-performing cows have led to a rising tide of infertility. Conception rates have fallen dramatically, chiefly because the over-worked animals cannot meet the huge physical demands made on them.

In the early weeks of each lactation they are expected to produce up to fifty litres of milk every day. In an instinctive drive to meet their genetically-programmed targets (i.e. the large amounts of milk they are bred to produce) they 'milk off their backs', in the old farming expression, metabolizing their own body tissues and diverting the products into milk. At the same time they are expected to get into calf again. Not surprisingly many fail to achieve it.

The excessive breakdown of body tissue clogs up the liver with fat. Hormone secretion is disrupted and conception rates fall away. More often than not the highly stressed animal is labelled as infertile and sent off to market.

In the face of such abuse, it's not surprising that the average dairy cow is worn out early. Traditional breeds grazing naturally on herb-rich pastures for much of the year will remain productive for ten years or more.

Today many UK Holstein cows are sent for slaughter after just three years of milking. The chief reason given by farmers is that they failed to get in calf quickly enough. The sensible solution would be to return dairy cows to the habitat evolution prepared them for – open grassland – but the economics of modern milk production don't allow this. So an army of scientists is kept busy searching for technical fixes to the growing list of disasters resulting from industrial agriculture.

The current method of feeding cows is by a system called TMR – total mixed rations. All the ingredients that go to make up a cow's diet are blended together in a large, mobile mixing tub. The TMR is carefully formulated to keep the animal on her production target.

First there are fibrous foods or forages – mostly grass and maize silage – to keep the cow's digestive system in some sort of order. The mix will also contain energy-rich cereals and high-protein feeds to push up milk yields. Because these are mainly grown by intensive methods, dependent on chemical fertilizers, they're likely to be deficient in essential minerals. So an artificial mineral supplement is added to the mix.

TMR is the dairy technologists' answer to the problems of feeding the yield-freak cows they themselves have produced. The aim is to churn out the white stuff to a minimal quality standard at the lowest possible price.

A great deal of science goes into ration formulation. There's much discussion between farmers and feed company specialists about such things as energy density, starch-to-sugar ratio and the level of utilizable protein. The animals must be goaded into producing their fifty litres a day.

But what TMR can't deliver is milk rich in health-giving CLAs, omega-3 fatty acids, vitamins and minerals. This is the product of cows on their natural food – green plants – especially the fast-growing green grass of spring and summer. Grass preserved for winter in the form of silage cannot produce the CLAs of fresh pasture.

In May 2005, the dairy company Dairy Crest launched St Ivel Advance, an omega-3 enriched milk.[17] It was endorsed by Professor Robert Winston of Imperial College's Institute of Reproductive and Developmental Biology. On the Dairy Crest website, he warned parents that today's children were not getting enough omega-3 in their diets and he welcomed its availability in a user-friendly format. It was good advice. The supplementation of children's diets with essential fatty acids has been found to improve reading, spelling and behaviour of school children.[18]

There are benefits for the rest of the population, too. Omega-3 fats protect against heart disease and strokes, reduce joint pain and inflammatory conditions, and improve foetal development in pregnant women. The Dairy Crest marketing experts clearly believed the benefits of omega-3 fats were well enough known to stimulate a keen demand for their products.

Of course, you might wonder why milk needs to be enriched in this important nutrient. It's plentiful in the milk of cows that spend much of the year grazing in the traditional way. If cows were put back on good grass, the levels of omega-3 in their diet would rise along with vitamins, CLA and possibly many other valuable nutrients that the scientists have yet to evaluate. But livestock nutritionists have discovered that they can raise the omega-3 content of milk by boosting the levels of oils such as flaxseed oil or fish oil in the rations of housed cattle. So the cows stay in their sheds instead of treading the fresh green sward.

Under the present system, farmers are mainly paid on yield – the amount of milk, fat, and protein they produce. Though they get bonuses for keeping the bacterial cell count at a low level, there's little incentive to pasture-feed their herds and so produce truly high-quality milk.

On average, British dairy cows spend around half their lives on pastures. But this average includes a number of smaller herds still managed by traditional methods. At the other end of the scale are large herds whose cows hardly set foot on grass at all.

An increasing number of large herds are today kept indoors in steel-and-concrete cubicles for months on end. Inside their rations can be more carefully controlled. Why go to all the trouble of turning them out to grass when cheap, chemically-grown grains and industrial by-products will keep milk flowing into the tank?

The big dairy processing companies are adding to the pressures on natural production methods. On traditional farms cows calved in the spring so that the peak in the cow's lactation curve coincided with the flush of grass, and the seasonal surplus of milk could be turned into deep yellow butter, rich in antioxidants and protective fats.

In today's dairy industry the efficient running of processing plants has become more important that the nutritional quality of the product. The dairy companies understandably want to see their plants running at optimum capacity throughout the year, so they offer farmers substantial bonuses on the milk they produce in winter, when grass is hardly growing. This forces them to use larger amounts of grain, soya and silage in the ration.

While the scientific basis of healthy milk and dairy products is becoming ever clearer, the ruthless economics of modern milk production are driving farmers in precisely the wrong direction.

Early in 2004, the weekly farming paper *Farmers Guardian* featured the 'revolutionary' new milking parlour of a West Country dairy farmer. The paper reported that he had travelled to California to look at large-scale dairy farms. He had come back determined to set up something similar in the UK.

According to the report he now had a building big enough to accommodate up to 600 cows. The roof area totalled more than an acre and a half. Though it was made up partly of translucent panels – ensuring that the interior was very light – the building was equipped with 170 electric lights to provide round-the-clock daylight if needed. This was the result of American research, showing that extended daylight could increase milk production.

For high-yielding cows this vast new building was to be their entire world. While lower yielders were turned out to grass for a few weeks in summer, said the report, the top yielders were housed all year round. At milking time they simply walked from their cubicles to the central milking parlour and gathering yard. 'The new system has been designed around maximizing production and minimising labour input while maintaining high welfare standards,' stated *Farmers Guardian*.

Though all-year-round housing is still uncommon in the UK, many cows spend the greater part of the year shut away in buildings. And when they are out on grass in summer, it's a pasture very different from that grown on the traditional mixed farm.

The temporary grass 'leys' on which the cows used to graze were part of the arable rotation. After two or three years under grass the field would be ploughed up for wheat. Even though a pasture was only due to stay down for two or three years, the farmer would sow a mixture of grasses and herb species. It was considered important to provide grazing animals with a variety of nutritious vegetation.

As explained earlier in the book, a typical short-term ley might include several grass species – deep-rooting cocksfoot, Italian ryegrass for early growth, timothy and perennial ryegrass. In addition there would be two or three types of clover along with a number of deep-rooting herbs, such as chicory, burnet and the legume kidney vetch. Permanent pastures – grasslands that were outside the arable rotation – contained an even wider range of native grasses and herbs.

Through the 1950s and 60s, government farm advisors worked closely with fertilizer companies to cajole farmers into abandoning their species-rich pastures and relying instead on grass monocultures.

Modern ryegrass varieties – like wheat varieties – are bred to respond to high levels of chemical fertilizer. In 1950, British farmers spread just five kilograms of nitrate fertilizer to every acre of grassland. Today they are using twenty-five times as much with some using almost one hundred times more.

As chemical nitrogen rates went up, so the ryegrass monocultures put on more growth, allowing the farmer to keep more cows on fewer acres. No one worried too much about the nutrient content of the extra grass. Nor were they concerned with the effect on milk quality.

Next came a campaign to convert dairy farmers to silage making. Until the 1960s, most farmers made hay as their chief winter fodder crop. The chemical companies weren't happy with this. Hay meadows were cut just once a year and were rich in fertility-building clovers and wild plant species. They didn't need much fertilizer to produce a good crop.

Working with the government's farm advisors, fertilizer reps mounted a vigorous campaign to persuade farmers that they should rely on silage instead of hay. Silage – grown as a ryegrass monoculture – is cut two or three times in a season, and requires large amounts of chemical fertilizer.

Today Britain's flower-rich hay meadows have largely vanished, killed off by chemical nitrogen. Instead of hay cows munch grass silage in their TMR diets. Like chemical wheat from the arable fields, this 'forced' grass is depleted of minerals and vitamins. So the milk that goes into the farm tanker no longer contains its full complement of health-giving nutrients. Research has now shown that milk produced by cows eating hay contains more healthy omega-3 fats than the milk of cows on silage.[19]

Though it was British politicians who first began the process of ruining the nation's milk supply by introducing subsidies, it was the European Community that completed the job. Under the common agricultural policy farm ministers worked unstintingly to 'modernize' Europe's more 'backward' farms. This meant promoting large-scale industrial farming. Through the 1970s and 80s they offered dairy farmers huge grants and loans to enlarge their herds and put up vast sheds to house them in.

Alongside the grants they operated market support arrangements that consistently favoured large-scale producers and discriminated against small farmers. Long after the butter mountains and the milk lakes had become a political scandal, Britain's dairy farmers were being exhorted to increase production by shoving ever more starchy cereals into their overworked cows.

By the early 1980s the politicians knew that milk quotas were inevitable if Europe's growing surpluses were to be reined in. Milk quotas, when they came in 1984, heaped rewards on intensive farmers – those who had pushed their animals to the limit in the race for higher output. Those who had refused to farm that way – and who had maintained the health of their cattle by keeping them on forage diets instead of starchy foods – were penalized with lower quotas. Many never recovered and were forced out of business.

Today dairy farmers are getting out at an unprecedented rate. In the early 1970s there were 100,000 dairy farmers in Britain. Four out of five of them have now gone, and the dropout rate is increasing. By April 2004, there were fewer than

16,000 dairy farmers in England and Wales, a fall of 29 per cent in just five years. Among the casualties were some of the best farmers in the country.

Those that remain are turning themselves into factory-scale operations. Many modern dairy units are little more than a collection of industrial sheds, surrounded by acres of concrete and lit by security lights.

These are no longer farms. They are rural factories driven by the ethics of industry. The overriding aim is to drive down costs – to produce every litre of milk for the lowest possible price. 'Get bigger or get out' is the background refrain of bankers, accountants, management consultants and the vast army of advisors who have their own reasons for seeing farming behave like any other business.

To be fair, many dairy farmers feel they no longer have any choice in the matter. They feel they're being pressed like some gigantic Cheddar cheese. And turning the screw are the super-markets and the big milk processors.

A study by the Milk Development Council shows just who is making money out of today's commodity milk.[20] Over the decade to April 2004, prices received by farmers fell by a quarter. Prices to processors – the big dairy companies and co-operatives that buy milk from farmers and sell it on to super-markets – remained fairly stable. The big winners were the supermarkets, dominated by a handful of giant multiples – Tesco, Asda, Morrisons and Sainsbury's. Their margins almost doubled over the ten-year period.

In 2003, the retail price for liquid milk averaged 47 pence a litre. Of this, farmers received just 18 pence. The processors took 16 pence, and the big retailers 13 pence.

To stay in the game, dairy farmers pack more cows into their sheds, and constantly search for cheaper materials to feed them on. It's a game that has few winners. Farmers come under increasing strain while making little profit. Their long-suffering animals are goaded into producing even more milk, despite the toll in ill health, and consumers are supplied with products that are, at best, depleted in nutrients. The super-markets, by contrast, make bigger margins than ever.

What kind of culture is it that treats its food producers and their animals in so barbaric a way? When the villagers of the Loetschental Valley received the first butter of the season, they flocked to the church to celebrate and give thanks. In Britain the big retailers would be busy looking for ways to buy it cheaper.

John Webster, Professor of Animal Husbandry at Bristol University and Britain's leading expert on the welfare of dairy cattle, believes greater respect for the cow will lead to better returns for farmers.[21] It's no coincidence, he says, that Perrier water sells in his local supermarket for twice the price of milk. While Perrier is seen as an added-value product, milk is viewed

---

Threatened by low prices and cheap imports, Wiltshire dairy farmer Arthur Hosier took radical action. He began keeping his cows outside on his rolling chalk grassland for 365 days a year, even milking them outdoors in mobile milking units.

The measure dramatically cut his costs, enabling him to make good profits while other dairy farmers struggled to break even. What's more, the milk he produced was healthier than most other milk around. In a speech to the Farmers' Club in London he said, 'The milk produced from cows living in the open air is better in every respect . . . The milking outfit being moved frequently prevents the land becoming foul, and there is no need for expensive and palatial buildings.

'There is not the slightest doubt that milk produced under such conditions is of much higher feeding value than milk produced in stalls [inside]. It keeps longer, and is higher in butterfat. Infectious diseases of the udder are almost unknown.'

Hosier gave his speech in 1927. Then, as now, farmers suffered from rock-bottom prices and competitive imports. He showed that by producing healthy milk from pasture – and selling direct to the public – there were good profits to be made. Could such a policy help hard-pressed farmers today?

as a low-price commodity item. Yet is it any wonder that consumers see milk this way, he asks, when the dairy industry itself holds the same view – that it is a commodity to be bought at the lowest possible price?

Webster adds: 'There are good reasons why we should adjust our first priority for dairy farming from that of productivity at all costs to one based primarily on respect for the dairy cow and the land.'

Not surprisingly, the same social and economic forces that have downgraded British milk are at work in the United States. There, too, herds have got larger, cows are increasingly kept in 'confinement' rather than outside on pasture, small family farms are being driven to the wall. Food campaigners have had enough. They're intent on turning the tide, and the method they've chosen is modelled on a small revolution that took place in the UK.

In 1999, the Weston A. Price Foundation of Washington – a non profit making organization set up to disseminate the discoveries of the nutrition pioneer – launched 'A Campaign for Real Milk'. It was inspired by a group of English blokes who sat in a pub back in the 1970s and bemoaned the rise of the corporate brewers and the threat to British ale. Out of that meeting sprang the 'Campaign for Real Ale', the movement which saved traditional beer.

According to the Real Milk Campaign website, 'Back in the 1920s, Americans could buy fresh raw whole milk, real clabber and buttermilk, luscious naturally-yellow butter, fresh farm cheeses and cream in various colors and thicknesses. Today's milk is accused of causing everything from allergies to heart disease to cancer, but when Americans could buy Real Milk, these diseases were rare. In fact, a supply of high-quality dairy products was considered vital to American security and the economic well being of the nation.

'What's needed today is a return to humane, non-toxic, pasture-based dairying and small-scale traditional processing.'[23]

9
Revolution

In Japanese farmer Masanobu Fukuoka's book, *The One-Straw Revolution*, there's a picture of the author standing in a field of ripening barley.[1]

The crop looks thick and strong. Fukuoka expects it to yield as well as any in the district – perhaps in all Japan. This crop was grown without sprays or chemical fertilizers. And it's growing on land that hasn't been ploughed for twenty-five years.

To grow his crops Fukuoka simply scatters the seed on the ground in autumn. The seeds are sown in a standing crop of rice that's still a few weeks from harvest. A winter grain, such as barley or rye, clover seed, and the seed for next year's rice crop all go on the unprepared seedbed in autumn.

In early November the rice is harvested. Fukuoka thrashes out the grain and then spreads the straw back on the field to cover the newly-sown seeds and seedlings. After that there's no more work to be done until the early summer next year.

Through the autumn and winter the barley and clover seeds germinate and grow up through the straw mulch. In spring the rice seeds germinate and start to grow. In late May the barley is ready for harvest, a little earlier than if it were growing alone. Once more Fukuoka thrashes out the grain and returns the barley straw as a mulch on the growing rice and clover plants.

In autumn, when the rice is ripening, it's time to sow next year's seed by scattering them in the standing crop. And so the cycle begins again. Year after year the land produces two crops – a winter grain and rice. There's no ploughing or cultivating to do. No costly and damaging sprays or fertilizers are needed. Yet the yields are comparable with any chemical farm in the land.

To western eyes it seems almost too good to be true. In our experience food crops must be worked for, sweated over, protected with costly sprays, but here it's as if the land were providing something for nothing. That, according to Fukuoka, is exactly what the land will do if we allow it.

He calls his method 'do-nothing farming'. He also calls it 'natural farming'. Fukuoka – who trained originally as a micro-biologist – believes the term is appropriate, since his system works by 'co-operating' with nature rather than trying to improve on it through conquest.

The Fukuoka system relies on soil micro-organisms to prepare the soil, nourish the crop, and supply all the trace elements it needs. Clover is there to provide nitrogen by fixing it from the atmosphere. The all-important straw mulch gives the soil microbes the organic material they need to stay active.

The results – achieved over more than thirty years – give the lie to the agribusiness claim that traditional forms of farming are unproductive. When the Soil Association – which represents Britain's organic farmers – launched a campaign to highlight the danger of pesticides in everyday foods, they provoked a storm of protest from farming leaders.

One irate member of the National Farmers' Union wrote an equally irate letter to the weekly *Farmers Guardian* denouncing the Association's 'scare-mongering'. He accused the organic movement of wanting to 'go back to the Dark Ages and see a starving population'.

This is the common claim of modern agribusiness – that traditional forms of farming inevitably lead to food shortages. It's a myth. Across the world millions of people are fed well by methods that don't rely on the fertilizers, agrochemicals or the GM seeds of a few multinational companies.

Up until the Second World War, Japanese farmers practised highly-productive forms of agriculture, though for Fukuoka there was rather too much work involved. Like him, by careful timing they grew two crops a year from their fields – rice and a winter grain – but they also ploughed, applied compost and manure, and flooded their land.

After the war, the Americans introduced chemical agriculture to Japan. Although farmers produced no more food than before, they achieved it using far less labour. This seemed like a great advance, and soon all farmers had switched to the chemical system.

Fukuoka was horrified by these developments. He believed it should be possible to grow crops without chemicals, and with a lot less work than traditional methods demanded. He hit on the idea of how to achieve it when he saw healthy rice seedlings growing up through a tangle of weeds in a field that had been neglected for years.

He realized there was no need to flood the land to grow good rice crops. Seed could be scattered directly on the land, as happened naturally in the wild. And why bother to plough in order to get rid of weeds when they could be controlled with a permanent covering of straw?

'This method completely contradicts modern agricultural techniques,' Fukuoka tells visitors to his farm on the southern island of Shikoku. 'It throws scientific knowledge and traditional farming know-how right out of the window.

'With this kind of farming – which uses no machines, no prepared fertilizer, and no chemicals – it is possible to attain a harvest equal to, or greater than, that of the average farm. The proof is ripening right before your eyes.'

According to Fukuoka, the reason modern chemical methods appear necessary for food production is that the natural balance has been so badly upset by those same methods the land has become dependent on them. Nature, left alone, is in perfect balance, he says. Harmful insects and plant diseases are always present, but do not occur in nature to an extent requiring poisonous chemicals. The sensible approach to disease and insect control is to grow sturdy crops in a healthy environment.

His philosophy flies in the face of western ideas about agriculture, but it clearly works. He expects a yield of 22 bushels of rice and 22 bushels of winter grain – barley or rye – from each quarter-acre of land. In a good year the harvest for each grain can be as high as 29 bushels per quarter-acre. This converts to more than 6 tonnes per hectare in western agricultural terms. In 2004, the UK barley crop averaged 5.8 tonnes hectare for both the winter-sown and spring-sown crops.[2] The UK yield was achieved with the whole arsenal of chemical fertilizers, sprays and hybrid seeds, and, of course, there was no second crop of rice from the same land.

Fukuoka applies four cardinal principles in his farming system. First, there must be no cultivation – no ploughing or turning of the soil. The earth cultivates itself naturally, he says, by means of the penetration of plant roots and the activity of micro-organisms, earthworms and small animals. Secondly, no chemical fertilizer or compost must be used. If left to itself, the soil maintains its fertility naturally, in accordance with the orderly cycle of plant and animal life.

The third rule is there must be no weeding either physically or by the application of chemical weedkillers. Weeds play their part in building up soil fertility and in balancing the biological community. They need to be controlled, not eliminated. Finally, there must be no dependence on chemicals, he insists.

The same four principles are applied to the growing of vegetables. The traditional Japanese way of growing vegetables for the kitchen blended well with the natural pattern of life. In his book Fukuoka explains:

Children play under fruit trees in the backyard. Pigs eat scraps from the kitchen and root around in the soil. Dogs bark and play, and the farmer sows seeds in the rich earth. Worms and insects grow up with the vegetables. Chickens peck at the worms and lay eggs for the children to eat.

The typical rural family in Japan grew vegetables in this way until not more than twenty years ago.

Plant disease was prevented by growing the traditional crops at the right time, keeping the soil healthy by returning all organic residues and rotating crops. Harmful insects were picked off by hand, and also pecked by chickens. In Southern Shikoku there was a kind of chicken that would eat worms and insects on the vegetables without scratching the roots or damaging the plants.

Some people may be sceptical at first about using animal manure and human waste, thinking it primitive or dirty. Today people want 'clean' vegetables, so farmers grow them in hothouses without using soil at all. Gravel culture, sand culture and hydroponics are getting more popular all the time. The vegetables are grown with chemical nutrients and by light, which is filtered through a vinyl covering. It is strange that people have come to think of these vegetables grown chemically as 'clean' and safe to eat. Foods grown in soil balanced by the action of worms, micro-organisms and decomposing animal manure are the cleanest and most wholesome of all.[3]

To describe this kind of farming as 'unproductive' is crazy. Far from taking the world back to a new Dark Age, it could be producing healthy, nutrient-rich foods from an unpolluted countryside. This is a fact denied by the captains of agribusiness with chemicals to sell. They portray traditional farming as quaint, picturesque and hopelessly impractical.

As a result the peoples of the wealthiest nations on the planet continue to eat third-rate food.

Fukuoka had rediscovered a secret known to many primitive peoples – that the land can be bountiful when natural laws are respected. It's a discovery that farmer Newman Turner made in the years following the Second World War. Chapter 6 explains how Turner used natural methods to control animal disease. He also found it was very profitable (see box).

When he took over as manager of Goosegreen Farm in Somerset during the Second World War, Newman Turner had unashamedly used every pound of chemical fertilizer he could lay his hands on.[4] But he struggled with diseased animals and crops, and the farm made a massive trading loss even though wartime prices to farmers were high.

So he gave up using chemicals or the plough. Instead he decided he would work *with* nature. He sowed his cereal crops into soils that had been cultivated with disc harrows. If there was too much weed or stubble 'trash' on the surface for the seed drill to work properly, he scattered the seeds on the surface ('broadcast' them), just as Fukuoka had done.

He soon started to harvest bumper crops. Following an unusually dry summer in 1948, for example, his wheat crop yielded almost 5 tonnes per hectare. Modern wheat growers would expect to harvest 8 tonnes a hectare in a 'normal' season, but only after applying a battery of fertilizers, pesticides and growth regulators. More than half a century ago Turner was achieving two-thirds as much with scarcely any inputs. There were no expensive sprays and fertilizers to pay for. Neither were he or his staff spending long hours on the tractor, ploughing, cultivating and working the land to get a fine seedbed. The UK average wheat yield in the early 1950s was just 3 tonnes a hectare.[5]

For his pasture fields he included clover and deep-rooting herbs in his grass seeds mixture. The clover supplied nitrogen while the herbs brought up minerals from deep down in the subsoil. On these mineral-rich pastures, the herd of pedigree Jersey cows stayed healthy and productive, and Turner's milk sales rose steadily. During the war – when he had used chemical fertilizers – half the cows had been infected with TB, calf abortions were running out of control, and the herd had been losing nearly £3,000 a year. By 1950 it was making a profit of over £2,000 – worth £120,000 today.

The cows had recovered their health – many lived for twenty years or more. They grazed the herb-rich pastures most of the year, so it's likely the milk would have been of the highest nutritional quality, high in vitamins, minerals and protective fats. This quality of milk is difficult, if not impossible, to buy today.

Most farmers would deny that such achievements were possible without chemicals.

As an agricultural student in the 1960s, I was inspired by a book that was by then more than twenty years old. George Henderson's *The Farming Ladder* had been published during the Second World War.[6] It told the story of a small farm on the edge of the Cotswolds, and of the two city-born brothers who ran it through the tough years of the Depression between the two wars (see box).

When the book appeared in 1944, it became an immediate bestseller, selling in the tens of thousands and running to more than six editions. Many of those who bought it were young servicemen and women dreaming of a better life after the war, for *The Farming Ladder* showed how any hard-working youngster could make a good living from farming.

It didn't take a vast acreage. Nor did it take a huge amount of capital. When George Henderson and his brother Frank moved into Oathill Farm in the early 1920s they had only one aim – to raise the fertility of their poor, stony-brash soils. This they achieved by steadily increasing the number of livestock, and by returning all waste – from both animals and crops – to the land.

On their little farm they introduced almost every form of livestock, including cattle, sheep, pigs, hens, geese and working horses. And despite the number of animals, they also sowed a large area with arable crops each year, chiefly wheat, barley and oats. It was the ordinary British mixed farm, the sort you see illustrated in children's picture books. But there was nothing ordinary about its results.

As the copious amounts of animal manure built up the levels of humus and organic matter in the soil, so crop yields rose year by year. Within ten years the Henderson brothers had made enough money from their small rented farm to buy the freehold outright. Land prices were relatively cheap in the years before the Second World War, but even so it was a remarkable achievement at the end of the deepest farming depression of the twentieth century.

By the onset of the war, Oathill Farm had become so productive it was held up as an example to other farmers of how they could feed the nation during the U-boat blockade. A report by the local 'War Ag' (War Agricultural Committee, the official committee which took over the wartime administration of food production in each county) showed that, on a per-acre basis, the little Oxfordshire farm carried three times the cattle, four times the breeding sheep, ten times the pigs and twenty-five times the poultry of the average farm in the county. At the same time it had a higher percentage of its land in arable crops.

George Henderson was one of those farming fanatics that urban societies seem to produce from time to time. Though he grew up in London there was nothing else in life he wanted to do. From his earliest youth – he once wrote – he had believed 'there was only one thing worth doing on earth – farm it!'

Having taken a correspondence course in agriculture – and worked on a number of farms to gain experience – he went to the bank with an offer they could very easily refuse. It seemed a ridiculous idea. He wanted a loan to go into farming; this at a time when farm prices were tumbling, and established farmers were going bust. Here was a nineteen-year-old with no capital, proposing to start from scratch. The manager practically laughed him out of the door.

But the Hendersons weren't easily put off. They managed to borrow enough cash from their mother to cover the cost of the 'in-goings'. With a little over £200 in working capital they took over eighty-five acres of stony Cotswold brash in the spring of 1924, just as the farming recession was starting to bite.

The brothers had a master plan. They would adopt a system that had stood the test of time – mixed farming. What had been good enough for British farmers over a century and a half was good enough for them, but they would push the system to its limits. They would discover whether a farm based on natural biological cycles could also be an intensive farm.

With their small amount of capital they started building up the livestock numbers. They reared chickens in outdoor arks, watching them grow strong and healthy on fresh grass and the insects they found in it. They also reared geese on fresh green crops of grass, mustard and trefoil clover planted in the corn stubbles.

As poultry numbers grew, they took to rearing young pullets in fold units – portable arks with wire runs attached. These were moved daily to a fresh patch of grass or stubble. The rich manure left behind by the chickens helped to build up the soil fertility, laying the foundation of bumper crops when the time came to plough up the grass and sow cereals.

Next the brothers began building up a herd of pedigree Jersey cows, rearing up to twenty-five heifer calves a year for sale to milk producers. The cattle remained remarkably healthy. In twenty years of farming the brothers didn't suffer a single case of bovine TB in their herd, even though the disease was rife among dairy cows. Mastitis was another disease that never appeared at Oathill Farm.

As they accumulated more cash they expanded their flock of pedigree Border Leicester ewes until they numbered forty. The lambs were sold for meat or as breeding stock. Though the enterprise seldom made big profits, the Hendersons were glad of the sheep. After all, the sheep flock had been known as 'the golden hoof' through Britain's farming history because of the invaluable part it played in improving soil fertility.

There was another reason George liked having the sheep around. There was nothing to match 'the pleasure of seeing lambs playing in the spring sunlight', he wrote, 'running races up and down the banks of our clear-flowing stream, leaping over it, and getting such fun out of life as only lambs can.'

As if there weren't enough livestock, the brothers ran a

herd of twelve pedigree Large White sows on their little farm, selling many of the offspring as breeding stock and fattening the rest for bacon.

The pigs – like the other animals – remained largely free of disease. The piglets got off to a good start by being fed Jersey milk at weaning time. As older animals they were allowed plenty of 'green' feeds, such as kale, rape, vetches and root vegetables with tops attached. Breeding sows enjoyed a run of fresh grass growing on an increasingly fertile soil.

To modern farming eyes George Henderson's holding on the foothills of the Cotswolds must have looked like a scene from Beatrix Potter with its cows, sheep, poultry and pigs all sharing the same green turf. Henderson would have cared not one jot. He knew the fertility they brought to the soil was helping to grow cereal crops of up to 2½ tons to the acre, an outstanding yield for the time. Today's cereal growers might expect more. But they make precious little profit. Much of the return is swallowed up in the cost of chemical fertilizers and sprays without which there'd be no crop at all on their impoverished soils.

Any lingering doubts about the credibility of this little farm are quickly dispelled by a glance through the penultimate chapter of *The Farming Ladder*. In it George Henderson sets out the full farm accounts for three sample years. The figures for 1942 – the last full year before the book was published – show an extraordinary profit of nearly £4,500. At today's values that's equal to up to £500,000.[7]

Admittedly this was midway through the war, a period of high prices following lean inter-war years. But even in 1932 – the low point in the farming depression – Oathill Farm notched up a profit of nearly £600 – £95,000 in today's money.[8] Suggest to any modern farmer that there was money like this to be made from just 85 acres of less-than-ideal land and they'd laugh in your face. It's more than a farm ten times the size would be likely to make today – and that's with the taxpayer putting in thousands of pounds in subsidies.

It's no surprise that the Hendersons' farming system should have been so productive. Biologically it was far more diverse than today's specialist industrial farms with their monocultures and paucity of crops. Farms – like natural ecosystems – are likely to be more productive the more complex they are, as science writer Colin Tudge observes in *So Shall We Reap*.

> The mixed farm is the key to the future of all humanity. For when crops and livestock are judiciously mixed, agriculture mirrors nature, and nature works . . . Animals, plants, fungi and all myriad variety of other organisms complement each other, and feed off each other. Plants create organic material by photosynthesis. Animals eat plants, and return the materials to the soil in their manure, in forms that the plants in turn can feed upon. Fungi, bacteria, and other 'detritivores' mediate the interactions. This simple cycle is elaborated in myriad ways but this is the essence of it. The key issue is that of ratio: the right proportion of animals to plants.[9]

The Henderson brothers understood this essential relationship between plants and animals, and adopted a farming system that made use of it. They weren't alone. At the time, tens of thousands of other farmers were doing something similar up and down the country. It was an ancient wisdom they had inherited. Not all of them did it as efficiently – or as profitably – as the Hendersons. But all were hard-working, resourceful and independent. And all were producing nutritious, uncontaminated food.

Today we'd probably think of them as 'food heroes'. That was the view of one contemporary commentator, the author H. J. Massingham, an astute observer of rural matters in the 1930s and 40s. In his book *The Wisdom of the Fields* he describes some of the small peasant farmers he met in the part of England where I live, the 'hillock and dingle country' between the Quantocks and the Brendons in west Somerset.[10]

There were the couple who grew enough food on their tiny smallholding – just four-and-a-half acres on the side of a steep hill – to feed a small village. Their wartime crops included strawberries, early and maincrop potatoes, orchard fruits, plus a greater diversity of vegetables than many a grower 'with four hundred acres of fat and level land.' In addition there were enough pasture, fodder crops and flowers to support a pony, over a hundred chickens, goats, ewes, a breeding sow and her litter of eight, and thirty hives of bees.

Not far away lived another couple with a farm of 75 acres. With the help of one woman worker – a girl from the wartime Land Army – they grew wheat, barley, oats, kale and root crops. They milked a herd of eleven cows, carting all the manure out to the fields. They also fattened sixty yearling sheep on root crops, corn stubbles and pastures. In six years, they had doubled the output of the farm, writes Massingham, as well as the fertility of their soil.

Before the advent of chemical farming, small, traditional farms like this were the mainstay of British agriculture. Then – as now – they were often portrayed by politicians and economists as backward and inefficient. Yet they cost taxpayers nothing in subsidy. And they supplied natural, healthy foods to local shops and markets.

A 1955 report by the independent policy group the Rural Reconstruction Association was in no doubt of the value of small, traditional farms. They were, according to the association, 'as efficient as large farms in the production of corn crops, rather more efficient in the production of potatoes and root crops, and markedly superior in the growth and utilisation of grass and *forage* crops.'[11]

George Henderson would have agreed. He compared the output of his small, traditionally-run farm with that of what he called well-managed, large-scale farms. He quoted wartime figures published in the *Daily Telegraph* for three well-known estates, ranging in size from 11,000 acres to 30,000 acres. Their outputs were one-third or less than that achieved by the Henderson brothers on their little Oxford-shire farm.[12]

Modern farmers become defensive at any suggestion that the food they produce is less than the best. At a farmers' conference, I was once almost lynched for suggesting the food I ate as a youngster in the 1940s and 50s was healthier and more nutritious than the foods on offer today. But the facts are inescapable.

As I reiterate in this book, before chemical fertilizers and sprays were freely available, farmers had no option but to care for their soils. Their business survival depended on it. The land had to be kept in good heart if there were to be crops to sell next year and the year after.

In the same way there was a real incentive to keep cattle healthy by giving them natural feeds and avoiding the overcrowding that might encourage disease. Before the advent of cheap antibiotics there was no other way to keep stock fit and productive. Almost by definition foods produced by traditional methods were healthy and nutritious.

Small, mixed farms, numerous at the end of the Second World War, had mostly emerged from the pre-war depression in good shape. The collapse of the international wheat price had taken a heavy toll of specialist arable farms, but the markets for beef, mutton, bacon, chicken, eggs, milk, cream and vegetables had all remained strong.

Back in the 1920s, farmers growing commodity grains for a global market had struggled to survive. But those growing nutritious foods for the people of their own country thrived.

Traditional mixed farming gave family farms a survival strategy through the bad years. And when food prices bounced back after the outbreak of war, they were able to enjoy better times. In *The Farming Ladder*, George Henderson urges farmers to use their new, wartime prosperity to 'put their farms in order' – to stock up with healthy, disease-free cattle and sheep. To depend on corn alone was to 'live in a fool's paradise', he warned.

Henderson believed the future for British farming lay with small-scale mixed farms. On a per-acre basis, he argued, they would always produce more food – and better food – than large mechanized farms. Only the small farm could achieve the necessary intensity of production by building up livestock numbers and returning all manure to the land.

He wanted to see the big landed estates broken up and split into small farms run by youngsters who, as farm-workers, had proved themselves capable. He didn't expect state handouts to finance them. They would work on profit-sharing farms while they built up the capital to take on farms of their own. As he himself had shown, there were plenty of profits to be made from well-farmed fertile soils, even in lean times.

He pointed to Ireland and Denmark as examples of the kind of farming he wanted to see. In 1923, the Irish Free State – later to become the Irish Republic – had begun buying up land from the big landlord-owned estates and selling it off to the tenants. The change had increased production per acre three-fold, said Henderson. In Denmark – a country similar to Britain – the farm output per acre had doubled during a period when the average farm size had been halved.

But if Henderson expected to see good farming and a prosperous countryside emerge in peacetime Britain, he had counted without the muddled minds of politicians. The government had taken a large measure of control over farming with the outbreak of war. The War Ags were given tough powers to tell farmers what crops they ought to grow – even to throw them off the land if their standards didn't come up to the required level.

The War Ags were generally unpopular, and most farmers expected them to be scrapped with the ending of hostilities. But the post-war Labour government of Clement Attlee had plans for the countryside. Under the watershed Agriculture Act the War Ags were to continue. The government also declared its intention to work for 'a stable and efficient agriculture' by means of 'guaranteed prices and assured markets'.

It was a piece of legislation that would sound the death knell for traditional mixed farming and undermine the whole basis of healthy food production. With the government guaranteeing prices for all the main farm products, there was no longer any need for balanced production. The more of a commodity you produced, the more money you picked up in state subsidy. It was simply a question of deciding which product to specialize in, then going flat out to produce as much of it as possible.

In place of mixed farming, large-scale specialist agriculture became the norm. Many farmers – especially those in the drier east of the country – got rid of their cattle and sheep, devoting themselves instead to growing monocultures of wheat or barley.

Soon the supply of manure began to dwindle. As a result, soil fertility started falling. But the new grain barons weren't worried, for help was at hand. The fertilizer companies had seen an opportunity denied to them in the pre-war days of mixed farming when farmers had been largely self-reliant. Soon the grain barons were relying on chemicals to maintain crop yields. This was more costly, of course. But public subsidies made it worthwhile. By 1960, just 1,000 large farms in eastern England were collecting more from the taxpayer than all 7,000 farms in hilly Carmarthenshire.

Livestock farmers, too, began re-inventing themselves as large-scale factory producers. As explained elsewhere in this book, this meant putting ever higher doses of chemical fertilizer on their pastures so they would carry two or three times the number of livestock. Along with the nitrate overdose came big sheds for housing the super-herds. There the healthy forage diet was diluted with cheap, chemically-grown cereals. In this way the taxpayers of Britain were duped into funding the degradation of their own food supply.

To George Henderson it was profoundly depressing to watch his fellow farmers and their leaders looking more and more to the state for help. For him the Agriculture Act of 1947 had been 'a crowning folly' in which farmers acquiesced to control by officialdom, bartering their right to farm as they pleased for an ephemeral guarantee of prices and markets.

He added: 'To invoke government assistance is like tying a brick to a cow's tail when she has flicked you in the face. The next time she swings it you'll be hit on the head with the brick.'

The destruction set in train by the post-war national government was brought to completion by the European Community. Through its common agricultural policy, the community, now the EU, has waged ceaseless war on good farming and wholesome, natural foods. The rules of the European subsidy system virtually obliged farmers to become large-scale specialist producers. Small farmers were offered bribes to get out, and large farmers were offered inducements to get even bigger.

There were generous capital grants for livestock farmers prepared to double the size of their herds. In the process many of them doubled the size of their debts and were forced to pile on more chemical fertilizers, and stuff more chemical grain into their long-suffering cattle.

On croplands there were handsome rewards for those who sprayed their wheat a dozen times through the season, then drilled the next crop almost as soon as the first had been harvested. The principle of balanced agriculture – with animals and crops together, as in the natural world – was consigned to history. So, too, was the idea of fertile soils based on organic matter and natural cycles. Farming was made an industrial process – a factory operation carried out in the open countryside.

The first farming revolution – the revolution of rotations and mixed farming – doubled crop yields and fed the nation during its emergence as an industrial power. The farming revolution of the twentieth century took away farmers' independence, ruined their soils and made the nation dependent on imported chemicals and oil for its food supply. And the foods themselves were degraded.

George Henderson warned that this kind of farming posed dangers for the nation. When Britain went to war it was the fertile mixed farms that were able to meet the demand for more food. He said that the large, specialist farms had been unable to cope. In *The Farming Ladder* he writes:

Large-scale farming in this country is the writing on the wall. When the guts have been torn out of land stimulated by artificial fertilizers, robbed by selling off all the produce, paying income tax on sales of straw which should have been consumed on the holding, then the farmer will be in the same position as an earlier generation after the last war. Declining yields and prices will complete his ruin.

But who would take a warning from me [he adds modestly], a fool who values his manure heap higher than his bank balance?[13]

10

The Fertility Furnace

Food shortages remained a real worry in early twentieth-century Europe, particularly for countries like Germany and Britain, where industrialization had been accompanied by rapid population growth. Farmers of the time relied mainly on organic wastes and legume crops, such as clover or beans, to return nitrogen to their soils and so maintain fertility.

There was also a thriving international trade in *caliche* – Chilean sodium nitrate, mined from the vast natural deposits on the arid plateau between the Andes mountains and the Pacific Coastal Range. This had followed an earlier boom in the mid-nineteenth century for guano, the nitrogen-rich sea-bird droppings from islands off the Peruvian coast.

By the turn of the century, the guano deposits had been largely exhausted, and it was clear that the nitrate-containing *caliche* would soon run out, perhaps in as little as twenty years. 'We are drawing on the Earth's capital, and our drafts will not perpetually be honoured,' the chemist Sir William Crookes had warned in his presidential address to the British Association meeting in Bristol in 1898.

During the second half of the nineteenth century, pioneer farmers had ploughed up vast tracts of the world's natural grassland to grow wheat for the industrial cities. South America, Australia and Russia had all yielded virgin grasslands to the plough.

Five years before the outbreak of the First World War, three of Germany's top chemical engineers made the journey from Ludwigshafen to the southern city of Karlsruhe, to observe a momentous laboratory experiment.

It wasn't an arduous journey. All three worked for the company BASF – *Badische Anilin- und Soda-Fabrik* – just sixty kilometres to the north. Even so, it would take something special to bring scientists of this seniority to the small lab in the physical chemistry department of Karlsruhe's technical university. At the time, BASF was the most powerful chemical company in the world.

In the lab the experimental apparatus had been set up on a bench. It was a compact and skilfully crafted piece of equipment made up of metal vessels, small-bore tubing and pressure gauges. Intrigued, the engineers inspected it carefully, though they had serious doubts that it could ever be made to work.

Its designer – a brilliant research scientist called Fritz Haber – had been emphatic. His process could harness the virtually limitless supply of the element nitrogen present in the Earth's atmosphere. In doing so it would free the world from famine, the scourge that had stalked mankind from the dawn of history.

At the heart of Haber's apparatus – which he called his 'furnace' – was an iron tube containing a nickel-heating coil. Inside the tube, a mixture of the two gases nitrogen and hydrogen would be introduced under pressure and heated to more than 500°C. In the presence of a suitable metal catalyst, the gases could be made to react, claimed Haber, forming the pungent white gas ammonia. What's more, the reaction would take place at a rate that made it a real commercial undertaking.

For BASF this was a prize beyond measure. Ammonia was easily converted to a soluble salt, such as ammonium sulphate, a valuable nitrogen fertilizer. The company that could find a way of producing it in quantity – and at a reasonable price – was on the road to riches.

As Chapter 5 recounts, the greatest transformation of all had taken place on America's Great Plains, and on the prairie lands of Canada. In a few short decades, the ancient prairie grasslands – haunt of vast bison herds and hunting ground of Native Americans – had been replaced, from horizon to horizon, by industrial grains.

For a number of years following the ploughing up of old grassland, crops produce good yields. They are sustained by the natural soil fertility built up under the turf, but after a series of wheat crops the land will eventually become exhausted. Unless some new form of fertilizer is made available in large quantities, the prairies, the steppes and the pampas will have to go back to grass.

In his Bristol address, Crookes set out the threat with the impeccable logic of nineteenth-century science. In the next century larger populations would need more wheat, he warned in sonorous tones. Yet there were few virgin territories left to be exploited. If the industrial world were not to go hungry, today's wheatlands would have to be induced to produce more.

It was Crookes who drew the scientists' attention to the vast reserves of nitrogen present in the Earth's atmosphere. Here was a way to feed the industrial masses. The 'fixation' of atmospheric nitrogen was essential to the progress of civilization.

This was a chemist's solution. Crookes concluded his address: 'It is the chemist who must come to the rescue . . . It is through the laboratory that starvation may ultimately be turned into plenty.'

Eleven years later the British scientist's challenge was about to be fulfilled in a laboratory in Karlsruhe (see page 156). That it should be happening in Germany was no great surprise. At the time the German chemical industry led the world. It was bound to be at the forefront of any new technical development.

There was another reason why Germany had a vital interest in cracking this particular nut. Antagonism between Britain and Germany was running high. To German military strategists it was clear that in any future conflict the Royal Navy would quickly block imports of Chilean nitrate, jeopardizing the nation's food supply. It would also threaten her military might. For nitrates were not just a valuable fertilizer – they were an essential raw material in the manufacture of explosives.

Without Chilean nitrate, Germany would be unable to fight a protracted war. The conversions of ammonia to nitric acid, and then to nitrates, were straightforward chemical processes. A limitless supply of ammonia derived from atmospheric nitrogen would add immeasurably to German military strength.

These were the imperatives that brought the three BASF scientists to Karlsruhe on that warm July day in 1909 (see box). It was a journey they made more in hope than in expectation. One of them – Carl Bosch – had already made a detailed study of ammonia synthesis. On joining the company as a young scientist, his first assignment had been to investigate the work of an earlier chemist who claimed to have produced ammonia from its elements. The claim turned out to have been mistaken.

While cautiously backing Haber's experiments, BASF had hedged its bets. The company had already invested in a Norwegian system for producing nitrogen compounds by passing electric sparks through air. This was a highly energy-intensive process. It could only make economic sense in a country with plentiful supplies of low-cost electricity – as in Norway. Even so, the company thought it a more promising development than the super-heating of gases under pressure.

If Fritz Haber entertained any doubts about his process, no one would have guessed it on that July day. He confidently pointed out the finer details of the laboratory apparatus. It included a number of innovative features. Research involving extreme temperatures and pressures threw up immense difficulties for scientists.

Many of those encountered by Haber were solved by his talented English assistant Robert Le Rossignol. Among the features designed by the Englishman were specialized valves to control the flow of pressurised gases, and a double-acting steel pump for circulating them.

For all its fancy design features, the apparatus almost failed on a simple engineering fault. One of the bolts in the high-pressure system sprang a leak during last-minute tightening. Producing a replacement delayed the experiment by several hours. Not until the afternoon was Haber able to open up the gas inlets and switch on the pump. By this time Carl Bosch was on his way back to a meeting in Ludwigs-hafen.

The two company men who remained were rewarded for their patience. Within minutes the first synthetic ammonia – now in liquid form – was beginning to rise in the water gauge. One of the two BASF engineers, Alwin Mittasch, turned to Haber and clasped his hand. He sensed this was a historic moment. And so it turned out to be.

Today most of the food we eat is grown with the aid of Fritz Haber's nitrogen. Around 40 per cent of the nitrogen in our bodies is derived not from the natural fertility processes of the soil but from super-heated gases in a steel chamber somewhere in Texas or the Ukraine. It has fulfilled the chemist's dream of making food plentiful and cheap, at least in the industrial countries.

As mentioned in Chapter 3, there's a dark side to the small, crystalline hailstones that agribusiness companies promote with such relish. They have become destroyers of family farms and rural communities. They pollute the seas and waterways. Worst of all, they have spoiled the foods of the countryside so they no longer promote good health.

Nitrogen fertilizers are a product of nineteenth-century industrial thinking. As a means of acquiring railways, roads and consumer goods, it has proved to be highly effective, but when let loose on the complex ecosystem of the soil it has taken us on a dangerous path.

After Haber's remarkable discovery, BASF put Carl Bosch in charge of developing the experimental process for full-scale production. He did it with a speed that was little short of extraordinary. The original bench-top converter had been just 75 centimetres tall. Four years later, an 8-metre high converter was producing more than four tonnes of

Once while on holiday in the Black Forest, I made a short detour to Karlsruhe. I wanted to find the building where Haber had carried out his historic experiment, if it still existed. It occurred to me there might even be some sort of museum with the original apparatus on permanent display.

I found the building easily enough. It looked no different from the pictures taken in the early 1900s. There was no science going on any more. The sign on the wall declared that it was now the Department of Architecture. I asked a couple of staff members about Haber's apparatus, but they couldn't tell me much.

Walking back through the old campus, I came across a piece of industrial art. On a stone pedestal had been placed what looked like an enormous metal cylinder – rather like the boiler of an old steam locomotive placed on its end. Then it dawned on me. I'd seen something like it in old photographs. This was the scaled-up production version of Haber's 'furnace' (the converter). The date on the accompanying plaque was 1919. The development of large-scale ammonia synthesis was as much a triumph of engineering as of science.

ammonia a day in the first commercial plant at Oppau near Ludwigshafen.

In another four years the company opened its second plant near the village of Leuna on the river Saale in Saxony. This one was capable of producing more than 100,000 tonnes of nitrogen a year.

By this time both factories were producing nitrates for Germany's war effort. Without them the German Empire might well have collapsed within months of the start of the First World War. It was only a steady supply of ammonia from the Haber-Bosch process that prevented the country from running out of munitions early in 1915.

Fritz Haber spent the war making another distinctive contribution to Germany's struggle. Following his success with ammonia synthesis, he had been invited to become director of the new Institute for Physical Chemistry, part of the Kaiser-Wilhelm Institute in Dahlem near Berlin. When war broke out, he turned the entire institute over to the development of poison gas. In the spring of 1915, he himself supervised the first gas attack of the war, releasing chlorine against French troops at Ypres.

At the end of the war he went briefly into hiding in Switzerland for fear of allied reprisals. Gas warfare was prohibited under the Hague Conventions. But far from being indicted for war crimes, he was honoured with the Nobel chemistry prize for his work on ammonia synthesis. It was a controversial award. Many scientists objected to the Swedish Academy's choice of 'the inventor of gas warfare'.

In his acceptance speech Haber declared: 'Nitrogen fertilization of the soil brings new nutritive riches to mankind. The chemical industry comes to the aid of the farmer who, in the good earth, changes stone into bread.'

Born in 1868 in Breslau, Prussia, Haber belonged to that eminent school of scientific rationalists who emerged in the late nineteenth century. Physics and chemistry were the dominant sciences. Haber combined the two with his interest in physical chemistry, and like most German scientists of his day, he made no distinction between science and engineering.

To him the job of the scientist was to provide practical solutions to society's problems. He was equally happy working on the efficiency of steam turbines, the thermodynamics of Bunsen flames or the extraction of gold from seawater. His role was to serve humanity – and, in time of war, to serve his country.

Nitrogen fertilizer is a product of that culture – of a nineteenth-century industrial mindset. From the moment the first ammonia dripped from the condenser in that Karlsruhe laboratory, industrialists around the world have been lining up to take it out into the countryside.

With the coming of peace in 1918, any hope BASF had of keeping the ammonia secret to themselves was quickly doused. Under the terms of the Versailles Treaty, the company was obliged to license construction of an ammonia plant in France.

Within a short time companies in Italy and the United States were building their own versions of the Haber-Bosch process, using what they knew about the basic principles.

In Britain, the chemical company Brunner, Mond had been producing ammonium nitrate by a variety of methods and was determined not to be left out of the race. During the war the company had worked closely with the Ministry of Munitions, running two Cheshire plants which produced ammonium nitrate by crystallization from sodium nitrate and ammonium sulphate.

In 1918 the government drew up plans to build a larger plant producing ammonium nitrate by the Haber process. A large site was purchased at Billingham near Stockton-on-Tees, but following the Armistice it was sold on to Brunner, Mond to develop.[1] The government also passed on all the details it had of the Haber-Bosch process, but crucial details remained a mystery. What were the operating pressures chosen by the German company? What catalysts were they using?

A team of Brunner, Mond chemists was dispatched to the Rhineland to study the processes used in the Oppau plant. They were accompanied by the assistant director of the government's explosive supply department, H. A. Humphrey. Under the Armistice agreement, German companies were supposed to disclose their industrial secrets. Even so, the Brunner, Mond board knew that without government backing the mission was a dead duck.

At Oppau, BASF managers were outraged at the spying mission, and did all they could to disrupt the visit. Production was brought to a halt, dials were hastily painted over and access ladders removed.

The 'spies' were banned from taking photographs or making notes. Whenever they walked into a production area, the staff would stop working and stare at the unwelcome visitors. Each night the British chemists would return to their hotel rooms and make notes and sketches from memory.

After a little over a month they thought they'd found out all they could. As they prepared to leave Germany, their baggage, including their report, was locked overnight in a railway wagon and placed under armed guard. This didn't stop a thief – or patriot – cutting through the floor of the wagon and plundering its contents.

Fearing such an incident, one of the team – a Brunner, Mond engineer called Captain A. H. Cowap – had kept his notes and sketches with him. Back in Britain they were enough to fill in many of the missing process details. For years afterwards the Oppau mission was referred to in the company boardroom as 'the burglary'.[2]

Thanks to this early industrial espionage, the Billingham ammonia plant was finally completed in 1923. Three years later Brunner, Mond merged with Nobel Industries and two other chemical companies to form Imperial Chemical Industries, ICI. Its first chairman – Sir Alfred Mond, later Lord Melchett – saw it as his mission to spread artificial fertilizers, not only across Britain, but throughout the Empire. Crucial to the enterprise would be propaganda.

Two run-down farms were bought near Maidenhead in Berkshire, one of which was called Jealott's Hill. They would become the company's research centre, along the lines of Rothamsted, the widely-respected Hertfordshire research station, which had been founded by an earlier fertilizer manufacturer, John Bennet Lawes. Jealott's Hill was to be the proving ground of the new nitrogen fertilizers. It would undertake serious scientific research to back up the marketing effort.

To give the company's research more credibility, an eminent scientist was needed to take charge. Mond persuaded Sir Frederick Keeble, Professor of Botany at Oxford, to become head of 'fertilizer research and propaganda'. He seems to have been well up to the task. After only four years research, he declared that the station had 'established beyond all question' how fertilizers could be used to increase food production and boost the fertility of farmland.[3]

Agriculture in the early 1930s was still sunk in recession. Keeble correctly identified the cause. Then – as now – farming stood exposed to global economic forces. New methods of transport meant that even perishable foods could be brought to Britain cheaply and efficiently. At the same time vast tracts of fertile, uncultivated land were being brought under the plough, especially in North America. British farmers were unable to compete.

Keeble had the solution. If farmers were to prosper in these stricken times, the fertility of the land – both arable and grass – would have to be raised. Only then would it produce more food; only then would it provide a decent profit for the farmer. And there was one obvious way of raising fertility quickly – through the liberal use of fertilizers.

Keeble was particularly keen to see livestock farmers applying the new nitrogen fertilizer to their grasses. He wrote:

> Nitrogen and mineral plant foods make grassland earlier, and more resistant to drought. They lengthen seasonal production, and convert the natural periodic exuberance into steadier growth. They increase the quality of grass as well as the quantity, and add to its health-giving properties. They give strength to the better grasses, encourage them to drive out the poorer, and so lead to permanent improvement of the grassland itself.[4]

Farmers weren't impressed. At the time they were applying a tiny amount of nitrogen fertilizer to their wheat crops – just five pounds to the acre. Hardly any of it went on grassland. Instead most farmers chose to rely on the fertility-building properties of clover. Despite the exhortations of Keeble and his colleagues, they had no intention of spending what little cash they could spare on chemicals.

With cheap grain pouring into UK ports from the American prairies, the response of many farmers was to get out of grain and put their fields down to pasture. Milk, poultry, vegetables, beef and sheep meat, as we have seen, all did well between the wars. Farmers found they could survive the recession perfectly well without ICI's fertilizers.

With unsold stocks piling up outside the Billingham factory, the company had no option but to shut down a large part of the plant. The budget for Jealott's Hill research station was cut by half, and shortly afterwards Keeble retired a disillusioned man. Propaganda had failed. ICI had set out to become the farmer's friend. Unfortunately the farmer didn't want to play.

The company had to find another way to spread the new chemical culture across the countryside of Britain. Instead of appealing direct to farmers, the decision was made to concentrate on influencing the government. If policy-makers could be made to see that chemical fertilizers were in the national interest, then they would do the marketing. The new strategy was given a shot in the arm by the outbreak of war.

Shortly before the war, ICI's chief agricultural adviser, William Gavin, had joined the Ministry of Agriculture. So the company already had its man on the inside. He and his former ICI colleagues began pressing the government to adopt a set of radical farming measures, 'in the national interest'. The main measures involved putting a lot of nitrogen fertilizer on grassland.

Research at Jealott's Hill had shown that an early application of nitrogen stimulated pastures to put on a spurt of growth in the early spring, so extending the grazing season. Other experiments had shown that silage – fermented grass – was a more reliable form of winter fodder than hay, the crop most farmers relied on. Needless to say, silage-making required far heavier inputs of nitrogen fertilizer than haymaking.

In the spring of 1940, the company mounted a vigorous lobbying campaign. They wanted the government to set national targets of a million acres of early grazing, and two million acres of silage. The extra grass would lead to enormous savings in imported cattle feed, they claimed, reducing the pressure on a merchant fleet that was daily running the gauntlet of Atlantic U-boats. What the company failed to stress was that the programme would require up to 200,000 tons of ammonium sulphate fertilizer.

At the start of the war the government was unconvinced. ICI chairman Sir Harry McGowan went as far as rebuking the agriculture minister – Reginald Dorman-Smith – in *The Times* for failing to set a clear farming policy. When Winston Churchill formed his government in May 1940, the new minister – R. S. Hudson – seemed far more compliant.

He announced a campaign for a million tons of silage to be run by the 'War Ags' that now controlled farming. They would rely heavily on help and support from ICI, the minister declared.

The following year Hudson approached the ICI chairman – 'my dear Harry' – for help with a wider campaign of grassland improvement to run alongside the silage programme. He appealed for the help of company staff to train and work with the government advisors. McGowan promised to help 'in every possible way'.

In the House of Lords, the government's spokesman on agriculture – the Duke of Norfolk – was forced to deny connivance with the powerful chemical industry. He added: 'There is no evidence that a balanced use of fertilizers has a harmful effect on soil, crops or man.' Nor, he candidly admitted, did it do any harm to ICI's profits.[5]

The company's plan to change the farming culture had worked like a dream. Before the government took on its emergency wartime powers, farmers showed they were uninterested in nitrogen fertilizers, particularly for use on grass. Once the war started they had no choice but to comply. The War Ags had absolute powers to control the way farms were managed. They could even throw families off their own land if they didn't do what they were told.

Not surprisingly, farmers started making more use of chemical fertilizers. The threat of invasion had set Britain on the path to industrial farming. ICI's own wartime campaign had been a textbook example of how to manipulate the British political system.

In peacetime the unholy alliance went from strength to strength. As set out earlier, the post-war Labour government introduced guaranteed prices for all the major farm commodities. For the fertilizer manufacturers this was a triumph. The state was contracting to pay farmers for whatever they could deliver. The message was clear. It was output that mattered, not quality.

This was exactly what Keeble had been calling for in 1930. Forget traditional methods, he had urged farmers. There was profit to be made by using chemical fertilizers to give a quick boost to production. At the time farmers had been sceptical. Now here was the government introducing the price guarantees to make it happen.

And in case there should be any confusion about the government's intentions, the new price guarantees were backed by special subsidies on fertilizers. The politicians and the chemical manufacturers were now on the same mission.

The state-run National Agricultural Advisory Service (NAAS), which replaced the county War Ags, swamped the countryside with meetings, farm demonstrations, discussion groups, all promoting fertilizers, especially nitrogen fertilizers. The chemical companies – most notably ICI – were doing the same thing. Many farmers believed that NAAS was simply a division of ICI. Others thought ICI was part of the government.[6]

The company was more than happy with the confusion. Endorsement by the official advisory service lent authority to the sales pitch. An advisory booklet for dairy farmers jointly published by ICI and the government-funded Grassland Research Institute had cover and illustrations printed in familiar 'ICI blue'. A popular saying with farmers was that the best grass seed came out of 'the blue bag' – the ICI fertilizer bag.

All these events took place fifty or more years ago. Yet the stranglehold of the chemical industry on the production of everyday foods is as tight as ever. Fritz Haber's breakthrough came out of the science of the nineteenth and early twentieth centuries – the age of industrial chemistry. In the rest of the economy it's a science that has been in steep decline. Today is the age of micro-electronics and biotechnology.

As Colin Tudge puts it in *So Shall We Reap*: 'In agriculture, though not in most of the rest of the world's economy, the glory days of industrial chemistry continue, confident and insouciant as ever'.[7] The farmers who once refused to put Haber's nitrogen on their pastures now throw it down at the rate of more than 100 kilograms to the hectare. Wheat growers on some of what used to be the world's best soils now find it necessary to use the world's highest rates of fertilizer nitrogen.

Generations of British farmers have grown up believing it's impossible to grow a decent crop without a bag full of chemicals and half a dozen pesticide sprays. Organic farming is seen as odd, chemical farming as the norm. It's as if agriculture had no history before 1940. This is how effectively a handful of politicians and industrialists succeeded in changing rural culture.

Even as the fertilizer manufacturers were getting their hands on the levers of power, Sir Albert Howard was warning of the catastrophe that would follow. In *England and the Farmer*, he forecast that the widespread use of artificial fertilizers would be condemned by history as 'one of the greatest misfortunes to have befallen agriculture and mankind'.[8] The crops they grew were poorly-nourished, so they had little resistance to disease. Nor would the animals and people that ate them.

Despite the warnings, Europe's farm policymakers made the same mistake as Britain's post-war government. They, too, put inflated prices at the heart of farm policy. For more than fifty years, Europe's farmers have been paid handsomely to maximize production with the aid of Haber's nitrogen. Much of the tax paid by Europe's citizens to support agriculture ended up swelling the profits of chemical companies.

Subsidies encourage farmers to produce more, which leads to higher prices for chemicals, seed, fertilizers, land and all the other inputs and resources they use. Only about a quarter of the subsidy ends up in the pockets of farmers – and then only the big operators.[9] The rest is paid out by farmers to supply companies, such as those providing fertilizers and pesticides, and in higher rents and land charges.

Only since 2005 have production subsidies been finally scrapped – too late to protect the health of generations of Europeans.

Today nitrogen fertilizers have become an international commodity traded, like oil, around the globe. A large part of the world's synthetic ammonia capacity is owned or controlled by energy companies. Because the process is so energy-intensive, most ammonia plants are situated in regions rich in natural gas, such as Siberia, Central Asia, the Middle East and the southern United States.

Ammonia synthesis now supplies about half the nitrogen used in crop production around the world. The biggest expansion came during the 1960s and 70s with the development of short-strawed, high-yielding varieties of wheat and rice (see page 73). Their use in Asia (especially India) became known as 'the Green Revolution'.

Many of the 'dwarf' varieties were bred by seed companies owned by chemical manufacturers. They had the great advantage of using large amounts of chemical nitrogen.

Norman Borlaug, winner of the Nobel Peace Prize and an architect of the Green Revolution, said that 'if the high-yielding wheat and rice varieties are the catalysts that have ignited the revolution, chemical fertilizer is the fuel that has powered its forward thrust.'

While the revolution has boosted the world supply of edible protein and energy, the crops it produces are depleted in minerals and antioxidants. Industrial agriculture is designed to produce large amounts of second-rate foods. It's these that dominate world markets, driving down prices and making it impossible for traditional farmers to compete. In rich countries and in poor, family farms are driven out of business by Haber's nitrogen.

When Sir Frederick Keeble was enthusiastically promoting ICI fertilizers in 1930, he promised farmers that the new chemicals would become their passport to a better future. Fertilizers would lift their output, he assured them, and secure them a better income.

In reality, the very opposite is true. Chemical companies have put them on a treadmill, forcing them to produce more and more to stay afloat. Colin Tudge sees the Haber-Bosch process as a highly-significant step on the path to industrial farming.

Before Haber and Bosch, fertility had mostly been a matter for farmers themselves . . . Farmers decided whether to grow clover, and how to balance stock against crops. Now the single greatest input (apart from water and sunshine and air) came courtesy of the fertilizer factory. Food processing and distribution were already well on the road to industrialization by the start of the twentieth century, but the production itself was not. After Haber and Bosch, the entire food supply chain had been brought within the purlieus of industry; and in particular, the chemical industry was firmly on board.[10]

Geographer Vaclav Smil believes the world's dependence on Haber's nitrogen is absolute, and there's no way back. Without it, he says, there's no way of maintaining high yields from most of the world's farmland. They now provide up to 80 per cent of the nitrogen used to grow the main food grains, such as rice, maize and wheat.

In his book *Enriching the Earth* – a review of the achievements of Haber and Bosch – he estimates that 40 per cent of the people now in the world are alive only because of ammonia synthesis.[11] The dependence is greatest in China, where political mismanagement of agriculture under the regime of Mao Tse-tung led to the worst famine in human history.

Following the opening up of China to world trade, the country placed orders for thirteen of the world's most modern plants for synthesizing ammonia and converting it to urea for fertilizer. In 1979, China became the world's largest user of nitrogen fertilizer, and a decade later it became the world's largest producer. Today two-thirds of the nitrogen in China's agriculture comes from Fritz Haber's furnace.

The United States is also a large user and producer of fertilizer nitrogen. But while China relies on it to keep its population alive, America uses it to keep its people eating large amounts of steak and its farmers exporting vast amounts of grain. About 70 per cent of US grain production is fed to livestock.

The world pays a high price for its acceptance of cheap food produced from synthetic ammonia. Quite apart from the health burden, there's a heavy environmental cost.

Only half the nitrogen fertilizer spread on the world's farmland gets taken up in crops. The other half escapes to the wider environment, where it frequently plays havoc with natural ecosystems. Much of it damages soil structure, leading to disease in crops and the disruption of microbial activity.

Nitrates leaching from farmland pollute rivers, streams and lakes across the globe. By the early 1990s more than one in ten of Europe's rivers had nitrate levels above the official maximum contaminant limit. High nitrate levels have been found in water wells throughout the American Midwest for more than twenty years.

Nitrogen enrichment of streams, lakes and estuaries encourages the growth of algae. When they decompose they take oxygen from solution, leading to the death of many aquatic species. The worst-affected offshore area in North America is in the Gulf of Mexico. Every spring, eutrophication by nitrates produces a huge toxic zone, which drives away fish and kills many bottom-feeding species.

The nitrogen fertilizer industry now puts into the world's life systems as much reactive nitrogen – nitrogen that is chemically active, unlike nitrogen gas in the atmosphere – as all the Earth's natural processes. Human interference in the global nitrogen cycle is now at a far higher level than for either the carbon or sulphur cycles.

No one can predict the environmental consequences. But the impact on food quality is all too clear. Our food is poorer. So is our health.

11
Back to the Sea

In the summer of 1977, ecologist and environmental campaigner John Hamaker (see Chapter 2) planted a small corn (maize) crop on a few acres of land he owned in Michigan. He described the land as 'worn out'. But before planting the corn, he 'mineralized' the soil by mixing in glacial gravel screenings – glacial dust – from a nearby quarry.

Hamaker, who originally trained as an engineer, had developed a theory accounting for climate change and the rise in atmospheric carbon dioxide. The Earth's soils were almost totally 'de-mineralized', he believed. The minerals that enriched soils, following the retreat of the glaciers 10,000 years earlier, had all but disappeared, leached away by rains and weathering.

On the now impoverished land, plants were no longer able to grow as prolifically as they had in prehistoric times. So the carbon that had once been locked up as organic matter in deep, fertile soils had been mostly lost to the atmosphere as carbon dioxide.

It was vegetation, coupled with the activity of soil microorganisms, that Hamaker realized regulated carbon levels in the atmosphere, but only for as long as there were adequate levels of minerals in the soil. When these were gone – as most have now – plants and microbes could no longer grow and multiply as they should. The stage was set for a new period of glaciation.

The theory also explained the rise in degenerative diseases. Hamaker was convinced that the loss of minerals from American soils was the prime cause of a catastrophic decline in the nation's health. In 1900, Americans had been judged to be the healthiest people on the planet. By the late 1970s, they were close to the bottom of the league table of the hundred healthiest countries.

It was to put his theories to the test that Hamaker applied glacial dust to part of his ten-acre holding in Michigan. Once the dust had been spread, he ploughed the land. In this way, the dust was mixed with soil to a depth of several inches.

When it was harvested the yield of the crop worked out at 65 bushels an acre. It had been a dry season, and conventional chemical farmers in the area were harvesting just 25 bushels with the same variety.

Even more impressive was the nutrient content of the mineralized crop. Hamaker had it analysed by a Detroit laboratory. They measured the major plant elements as well as protein content. Compared with a chemically-grown crop, the maize contained 57 per cent more phosphorus, 90 per cent more potassium, 47 per cent more calcium, and 60 per cent more magnesium.[1]

The protein content was 9 per cent, a high figure for hybrid maize. The more usual figure for protein is between 6 and 8 per cent.

Though the full range of essential elements were not analysed, there's little doubt that they, too, would have been high. Trace elements are essential for the thousands of enzymes that go to produce plant protein. If the protein level was high, the minerals must have been there to produce it.

In his book *The Survival of Civilization*, Hamaker wrote:

If the enzymes are not present, the protein cannot be produced, and the total protein level falls. That has been happening to US crops over a number of decades. So it's not surprising that all our livestock and a quarter of our people are too fat.

Neither is it surprising that so many handicapped babies are being born to mothers suffering from malnutrition. As the various elements required by enzymes disappear from the soil, body functions must inevitably fail, so that the diseases of malnutrition become the norm rather than the exception.

Hamaker found plenty of other examples of extraordinary plant growth following soil mineralization. An old organic

John Hamaker's colleague, Donald Weaver, tells the story of an intensive farmer in Vermont, whose father managed the local gravel pit. He ploughed in gravel screenings in an attempt to improve the drainage on a waterlogged section of the farm. The first crop grown on the mineralized land was clover. By the time cold, autumn weather halted their growth, the plants had reached 12 feet in length. The stalks were so thick and tough that the farmer had difficulty cutting them back with a set of disc harrows.

The following year the farmer grew carrots and broccoli on this part of his land. He later reported that the carrots reached a foot-and-a-half in length, while the broccoli head averaged two-and-a-half pounds in weight. All were grown without chemical fertilizers or pesticides.

Weaver was so impressed that he treated his own California garden with screenings from gravel pits east of San Francisco Bay. Afterwards, runner beans climbed to eighteen feet, before being turned back by the heavy weight of beans at the top. Weaver later reported that the flavour of the beans – along with the taste of lettuce, carrots, courgettes, cucumbers and melons – was 'wonderfully sweet and rich, shouting the story of an end to malnutrition and disease.'

garden was treated with mineral-rich glacial gravel. Afterwards a squash plant grew so big that it climbed all over a nearby tree, making it look like a squash tree.

Shortly afterwards, the owner decided to sell the property and neglected the garden. Before long weeds that would normally grow to two or three feet had shot up to eleven feet or more on the mineral-enriched land.

Another gardener – who happened to be the owner of a gravel pit – dug in the 'screenings', or dust, from the rock crusher. Soon the land was growing potatoes weighing three pounds each. In his own mineralized garden, Hamaker grew carrots that reached three inches in diameter and weighed a pound and a half.

As Chapter 2 explained, the stories have now found their echo in the Scottish Highlands, where Moira and Cameron Thomson grow large and flavour-filled vegetables in their 'rock dust garden'. Like the American farmers and growers, they have reproduced the fertile conditions that followed the retreat of the glaciers. For those mineral-rich soils to occur naturally, there would have to be another ice age, with glaciers to grind down a new crop of mineral-rich volcanic dust from rock.

Hamaker recommended the use of finely-ground glacial gravel for re-mineralizing a worn-out soil. This is the rocky debris left behind when glaciers retreat at the end of successive ice ages. The virtue of glacial gravels is that they're likely to contain fragments of a variety of rock types and so supply the full-spectrum of minerals.[2] The important thing is to use rocks of volcanic origin like those that make up the Sidlaw Hills in Perthshire, from where Cameron and Moira Thomson get their rock dust supplies. They use basalt, an igneous rock, in a dust fine enough to pass through a five-millimetre sieve.[3]

Hamaker's claim was that the world didn't need to wait for the catastrophe of a new ice age. There was plenty of mineral-rich dust lying around in quarries across the world. By spreading it on the land, farmers could re-awaken their soils and at last start to realize the full potential of their farms.

Re-mineralization could raise the output of farmland by up to four times, he argued. And the mineral-rich foods flowing from it would begin to reverse the tide of ill health that currently engulfed western societies. But first it would be necessary to break the stranglehold of the chemical industry on food production.

Eighty years or so before John Hamaker began campaigning on the health benefits of finely-ground rock dust, an earlier convert was doing battle with the fertilizer companies. In 1893, the German scientist Julius Hensel brought out his book *Bread From Stones*. In it he showed that a mixture of ground stones – representing a range of rock types – could produce high yields of crops rich in minerals.[4]

After much research Hensel claimed that his stone meal grew bigger crops, resistant to disease and strong enough to withstand drought and frost. The foods they produced were rich in taste and nutritional content, and seemed to improve the health of both the animals and humans that consumed them. In 1892, an exhibition was held in Leipzig of the foods produced by Hensel's stone meal, and plans were made to manufacture the material on a large scale. They were blocked by the absence of a commercial stone-grinding machine, and by growing opposition of those who took a differing view of food production.[5]

Hensel and his writings came under savage attack from the chemical interests of his day. They strongly supported Justus von Liebig's assertion that factory-made compounds of nitrogen, phosphorus and potassium were the best form of fertilizer (see Chapter 7). The few companies who tried to market 'stone meal' were forced out of business. Hensel's book – which contained testimonials from farmers who had successfully mineralized their soils with rock dust – was suppressed, and even removed from libraries.

Ironically, had Liebig – 'the father of agricultural chemistry' – been able to use the analytical equipment available now, he might have been less strident in his promotion of the three elements alone. His simplistic claims were based on analyses of plant tissues which showed the three to be 'major constituents'.

With modern equipment he would have discovered almost all the elements were present in plant tissue. The obvious conclusion to be drawn was that all of them should be supplied together in the form of finely-ground rock dust.

Liebig is the author of the famous Law of Minimum, which (in my day) was to be found in every school biology book. In his own words, the law states that 'by the deficiency or absence of one necessary constituent, all the others being present, the soil is rendered barren for all those crops to the life of which *that one* constituent is indispensable.' On this basis, chemical fertilizers with just a handful of plant elements could have been predicted to lead to trace element deficiencies and malnutrition.

Until pesticides began to be used widely, many British farmers relied on a by-product of the steel industry to remineralize exhausted soil. It went under the unprepossessing name of basic slag. During the conversion of iron to high-quality steel, the phosphorus present in iron ore had to be removed. This was done by blowing air through the molten iron to which lime had been added. The oxidized phosphorus combined with lime to form a scum which was poured off and solidified.

Finely ground, this material was used as a low-cost mineral fertilizer, rich in phosphorous that was made available to plants in the presence of the mildly acid compounds exuded from their roots. The lime in basic slag also provided a ready source of calcium, the key to a healthy, fertile soil.

The waste material had another benefit for farmers. It contained a wide range of essential minerals including manganese, boron, zinc, cobalt and magnesium. For generations of livestock farmers this by-product of steel-making returned health and life to worn-out grasslands.

In the second half of the twentieth century basic slag gradually fell from use, its decline linked to both changes in the steel industry and to the economics of farming. Some associate the collapse in the health of both crops and animals to its falling popularity. In the search for healthier crops soil specialists have now begun to rediscover its benefits. Among the new pioneers is Robert Plumb (see page 8), head of the Norfolk-based Independent Soil Services.

Plumb recommends basic slag wherever a full soil analysis shows it can help bring back life and fertility. He values the product for its unrivalled ability to restore calcium to healthy levels. Equally importantly, basic slag provides the trace element boron, essential in the metabolism of calcium. In addition, it contains selenium and manganese, elements that are as vital to the health and fertility of livestock grazing pastures as they are to the health of the people who eat the products.

Dusts aren't the only way of re-mineralizing soil. The world's oceans have long been known as a repository of trace elements. That's where the minerals leached from soils over the past 10,000 have ended up. According to nutritionist Bernard Jensen, 'trillions of tons' of trace elements, both known and unknown, reside in seaweeds, fish emulsions, kelp and other forms of sea life.[6]

In the United States, school children are taught that Native Americans on Cape Cod showed the early pilgrim settlers how to plant corn by placing fish heads in the rows for fertilizer.[7]

Jensen advocated the use of foliar sprays – prepared from finely-powdered seaweed – as a way of nourishing crop plants grown on mineral-deficient soils. In his book *Empty Harvest* he explains:

Trace elements such as iodine are rarely found in inland crops, but can be part of a healthy plant thousands of miles from the sea through foliar sprays. Trace minerals are absorbed directly into the leaf, and many insects are repelled by them.

I have twenty plum trees that have never produced bad fruit and never suffered insect damage. They were raised exclusively on foliar seaweed sprays, more than one thousand miles from the nearest ocean.

Another way of utilizing the elements found in the oceans is to extract them directly from sea water. Sea solids are designed to do the same job as rock dust – to replace the lost trace elements that centuries of weathering, and decades of chemical farming, have stripped from the soil. Former organic farmer, Oliver Dowding, supplies them in concentrated liquid form from his company Ocean Grown.[8] Farmers then spray them on their fields using the farm's own crop sprayer. With luck, the subsequent crops will be so healthy that the sprayer won't be much needed afterwards.

This form of re-mineralization is firmly established in the United States. It's based on the work of an American physician, Maynard Murray, an ear, nose and throat specialist (see Chapter 4). Like Ohio dentist Weston A. Price, Murray became alarmed at the amount of degenerative illness he was seeing in society.

In *Sea Energy Agriculture* (1976), he wrote:

> More than one hundred million cases of chronic or long-running illness and disablement afflict US citizens today. That's nearly half the population and many of these cases afflict the very young. These statistics are even more alarming if we take into account less disabling diseases such as dermatosis, chronic migraine headache and dental disease.
>
> Finally, the topping on the unsavoury morsel of medical fact is the distressing truth about infection. Despite our wonder drugs, steroids, sanitation standards and general medical wizardry, the United States has one of the highest infection rates per capita of any society.[9]

Chapter 4 mentions how Murray was struck by what appeared to be an absence of disease among sea creatures. He studied a range of marine mammals looking for the kinds of chronic decay that afflicted human populations. He found little. Nor could he find much evidence of ageing. He began to wonder about the reason. Was it some nutritional factor at play? He concluded that it was because of high mineral levels in sea water.

All soil minerals eventually end up in the oceans. As they leach from the land, they're carried down streams and rivers, and ultimately to the sea. Murray observed that sea water contained the elements of the Atomic Table in a solution 'of consistent balance and proportion'. In this form they were available to all marine life.

He also noticed that the elements in sea water were essentially the same as in human blood, and in very similar quantities. Was this a clue to the role of minerals in human health? Could mineral deficiencies be a major cause of degenerative diseases?

Following early success with sea water trials (see box), Murray began a series of experiments using 'sea solids' rather than sea water. These were produced by evaporating off the water as in the manufacture of sea salt, although greater care was taken to make sure the minerals left behind were in the same relative proportions as they were in solution.

In a long series of experiments, sea solids were tested on a range of crops, including maize, wheat, oats, barley, vegetables, clover and hay. All of them stayed healthier and produced heavier yields than crops grown on untreated soils. Chemical analyses showed they contained significantly higher levels of minerals, vitamins and sugars. Equally important, people eating the produce invariably judged them to have a far better flavour.[10]

In the early 1940s, the physician Maynard Murray embarked on a series of experiments to find out whether the minerals from the sea might be used to boost the levels in everyday foods. He started with undiluted sea water. The US Navy was called in to supply sea water from the world's oceans. This was carried in rail tankers to Murray's research site in Cincinnati. There he sprayed the sea water on trial plots, and planted a range of crops to see how well they would grow.

As part of the experiment, some were deliberately infected with disease. A turnip crop was infected with a bacterium associated with a condition known as centre rot. Though turnips in the control plots were spoiled by the disease, those grown on soil treated with sea water thrived. So did peach trees, which had been infected with a damaging disease known as curly leaf virus.

Garden vegetables, in particular, were 'superior' in taste. Onions, tomatoes, potatoes, sweet potatoes, apples and peaches were said to be 'outstanding'. The 'tasters' remarked that onions could be eaten 'almost as apples'.

Sometimes the taste panels were made up of animals. Maize cobs grown on land fertilized with sea solids were marked and mixed with chemically grown cobs, then fed to cattle on pasture. Murray was astonished to see the animals rooting through the heap and picking out the mineralized corn. The conventionally-grown cobs were ignored.

Even more extraordinary was the behaviour of sheep turned loose on a clover field, part of which had been fertilized with sea solids. The animals ranged aimlessly across the field until they reached that area that had been treated. They then stayed in that spot, grazing down the clover plants practically to ground level.

For many years, Murray worked with local farmers on a series of large-scale trials, looking at the feed value of mineralized maize, oats and soya beans. The results showed that both pigs and cattle remained healthier and grew faster when fed grains grown with sea solids. Chickens were particularly well-suited to them. Laying hens produced more and larger eggs; broiler chicken grew faster and produced meat of higher quality.

After more than 30 years' research, Murray published the results in his book, *Sea Energy Agriculture*. It was an urgent plea for a more natural approach to soil fertility, and a more nutritional approach to medicine and health.

He concluded:

American agriculture and food processing techniques
are attempting to accomplish the impossible – the me-
chanization of biology. In our driving ambition to produce more and more on less and less, we produce
enormous quantities of food of dubious quality. To
maintain high production rates in agriculture and animal husbandry, we resort to measures, some of which
border on insanity . . .

It is not difficult to see why our health is not good.
What is remarkable is that our health is as good as it is.
We are nutritionally deficient, and, as a result, we open
ourselves to attack from parasitic organisms. We submit
to slow poisoning through cumulative toxins, and try to
get something for nothing by defrauding nature. All the
problems inherent in our modern system can be eliminated with the application of sea energy in agriculture
and good sense in processing.

Murray's pleas fell on deaf ears and closed minds.
In the United States, nitrogen fertilizer was too big a business
to put in jeopardy. Led by the oil engineering firm
M. W. Kellogg Company of Houston, American engineering
firms were busy selling ammonia plants to China and other
countries around the world. The possibility that sea salt
might be enough to ensure high crop yields and healthy
foods was not a popular idea in chemical company board-
rooms.

On this side of the Atlantic, the UK had recently joined the
European Community with its farm regime of inflated prices.
Land values were escalating as city fund managers spotted an
investment opportunity in Britain's rolling acres. The way to
make money under the Brussels regime was to maximize
output with little regard for quality. Chemical fertilizers fitted
the bill admirably.

For the best part of half a century, the chemical industry has
effectively vetoed every attempt to re-mineralize over-worked

soils and restore the health benefits to everyday foods. They have perpetuated the myth that western countries must go on producing more and cheaper food, when the desperate need is for food that is more nutritious.

12
All To Play For

At first sight it's easy to be pessimistic about the future for real food. It's still there if you look for it. For a small, well-off section of the population with time to spare, there's good food on offer at farmers' markets and farm shops around the country. But for the majority of us who shop at supermarkets, most foods – including the so-called healthy options – are intensively-produced fakes.

The supermarkets themselves grow stronger by the day. Having established in consumers the habit of a weekly 'big shop' in the local superstore, they're now busy driving out corner shops by moving in with their pared-down city-centre outlets. They've even managed to 'dumb down' organic foods by restricting their buying to a small number of large-scale producers.

Out in the fields industrial agriculture appears as invincible as ever. Farms grow relentlessly bigger, and farmers seem obsessed not with the nutritional quality of their products but with turning them out at ever lower cost. As a nation we appear bent on self-destruction. We deny our bodies the nutrients they crave for, so we're left with more cash to spend on our homes and holidays.

At the same time there's a growing counter-culture trying to shift things in the opposite direction. Organic sales are booming. In newspaper and magazine articles, food writers decry the falling standards of everyday foods. Celebrity chefs and 'foodies' are becoming as concerned with the way food is produced as they are about preparing and cooking it. Following a seemingly endless series of food scares from BSE to Sudan Orange, there's clearly a rising groundswell in favour of real food.

But could such a movement topple the edifice of industrial food production, shored up as it is by so many powerful interest groups? It's starting to look possible, even likely. There are signs that Britain could be on the verge of a social revolution. It's not one that will fill the streets with banner-waving citizens, as in Eastern Europe in the late 1980s. This one will transform the rural landscape.

What's needed is leadership – from farmers, retailers or politicians. Large numbers of people are now dissatisfied with second-rate industrial food. They desperately want something better. But to make the choice they need to see real food on the shelves at a reasonable price, and they need to know how to identify it. They need the food, and they need the full story about how it's produced.

If it chose to, the government could make the necessary changes with ease. With sensible legislation it could bring real food within reach of the whole population, and, at the same time, provide a brighter future for family farms. Some would claim the politicians were under an obligation to act. After all, it has been ill-judged farm policies of 60 years that have robbed people of their food heritage, in effect, selling out agriculture to the chemical industry. But to take strong action now, government ministers would first have to acknowledge the mistakes of the past.

Politicians don't quite 'get' farming. If they think about it at all they see it as an activity much like the IT industry – an enterprise that must be forever re-inventing itself, constantly grasping at new technologies to be successful. This was once

As director of the Soil Association, Patrick Holden is one of the country's leading campaigners for better food. He's also a farmer, and on his organic farm in west Wales he has been growing organic carrots since 1979.

Organic carrots from Bwlchwernen Fawr near Lampeter started to appear in UK supermarkets twenty years ago. Patrick remembers Sainsbury's packing their first organic carrots in his cowshed. Through the 1990s he made good money from his annual field of carrots. But as the organic vegetable-growing became 'industrialized', production shifted from small mixed farms like Bwlchwernen Fawr to large-scale specialist operations in East Anglia.

These 'commodity' producers came to dominate the market, driving down prices to the point where growing carrots on small mixed farms became uneconomic. In 2003, Patrick decided not to plant his carrots, the first time he had failed to do so in twenty years. At the prices being offered by the supermarkets he could see no way of making a profit.

A year later he went back into the crop, chiefly because it suited the rotation on his mixed organic farm. But this time he was determined to grow them on his own terms and market them in a very different way.

He commissioned his daughter Barley – a teacher and a talented artist – to paint a picture of the west Wales farm. It shows the farmhouse and buildings set amid the rolling Welsh hills. In the foreground there's a bunch of carrots, their feathery green tops still attached.

With no guarantee of a market, Patrick then had the picture printed on thousands of polythene bags. Above and below it ran the brand label: 'Welsh Organic Carrots. Grown by Patrick Holden, Bwlchwernen Fawr.'

On the reverse of the bags he told the story behind the crop.

'Our 240-acre organic family farm rises to 750 ft in the hills of West Wales in a beautiful and unspoilt landscape', it reads. 'Our crop rotation starts with clover and grass, which feeds our sixty-five Ayrshire dairy cows, followed by carrots and oats. After more than thirty years of organic farming there is a strong impression of food production taking place in harmony with nature.

'We usually grow one field of carrots each year, of around

five acres. You will find a range of sizes and shapes as this is how they grow in nature. We oppose excessive cosmetic grading which often results in up to 40 per cent of the crop being wasted. We hope you enjoy their quality and flavour.'

Patrick offered his carrots and their new packaging to three major supermarkets. He told them what the price would be, and that he wasn't prepared to negotiate. They could take it or leave it. One of the supermarkets – Sainsbury's – agreed to stock them in their Welsh stores alongside their own-label organic carrots. These had been strictly graded, making them more or less uniform in size. They were also priced at 20 pence a bag less than the crop from the Welsh hills.

Patrick's carrots in their colourful, informative bags went on sale in January 2005. Within two weeks Sainsbury's had taken their own-label organic carrots off the shelves. Sales of carrots from the Welsh farm had beaten them hands down. When presented with a real food with a real story, shoppers were no longer interested in the cheaper, anonymous version, even though they were more strictly graded and had an organic label attached.

To Patrick the message is plain. Faced with a clear consumer demand the supermarkets will act very quickly. Never mind the economic trends of the past four decades; never mind the drift to industrial farming with its chemicals and monocultures. Once the supermarkets identify a growing interest in real, or local, foods these products will start appearing on the shelves almost immediately.

'Consumers have no idea how powerful they are,' Patrick says. 'They could change the food – and the landscape – of this country almost instantly. The major supermarkets are locked in a desperate competitive battle with each other. They are obsessed with giving consumers what they want. When they spot a new consumer trend they'll respond to it instantly. This gives shoppers a real opportunity to change the food system.

'It wouldn't even take many. A small number of shoppers demanding properly-grown food could spark a revolution.'

the view of the Prime Minister, Tony Blair. In a speech to the Royal Society he warned that without advanced technology – and in particular genetic engineering – the growing world population could not be fed. By implication anyone opposing genetically-modified crops was a romantic Luddite prepared to see half the world starve.

But according to the science writer Colin Tudge, this view is flawed. In his critique of industrial farming, *So Shall We Reap*, Tudge argues:

> Genetic engineering has so far contributed nothing of significant use in feeding the world. Its contributions have purely to do with ease of husbandry, and hence the reduction of costs.
>
> There is no good reason to assume that genetic engineering will contribute anything that the world actually needs within the next half century – in which time the world population will have stabilized, and the heat will be off.[1]

As I've pointed out at intervals throughout this book, industrial agriculture is the offspring of nineteenth-century 'reductionist' science. It works by looking at the effect of a single measure or action taken in isolation. This might be the application of a new pesticide or the introduction of a novel crop variety. Whatever the innovation, when it leads to an increase in yield, commercial farmers quickly grab it in their frenzy to produce more at lower cost.

In the biological world things are never that simple. In complex living systems like the soil, there will be a range of (sometimes subtle) effects. For example, a new chemical fertilizer may reduce the activities of soil micro-organisms which would otherwise make essential trace elements available to plant roots.

Such subtleties are ignored in industrial farming – until, that is, they begin to have damaging consequences. Then the 'agri-technologists' embark on a frantic search for some new technical 'fix'. In this way, the business of growing food is turned into one unending battle with nature.

In mainstream biology the reductionist approach has been largely discredited. Modern genetic research shows it to be a poor explanation of the way living organisms work. For years genetic scientists have searched for genes that might be responsible for conditions such as heart disease, schizophrenia and autism. But they've proved to be remarkably elusive. Rather than being 'caused' by particular genes, it seems these diseases are more often the result of small actions by a large number of genes.

The idea of the gene at the centre of living processes – a concept given credibility by the 'selfish gene' theory – has now given way to the view of the 'multi-tasking gene' operating as part of an integrated network. In response to this new way of thinking, courses in 'systems biology' are springing up on campuses around the world. In most of them physicists, mathematicians and engineers work alongside biologists in a network that mimics the natural systems they're studying.

In farming, the outdated reductionist view still holds sway. Agronomists still throw chemicals at crops and look for yield advantages. It's the chief reason for our spoiled food and polluted environment. Because it fails to account adequately for living processes, it seems destined to collapse.

The irony is that the traditional farming patterns adopted the same integrated approach as modern biology. By instinct traditional farmers recognised that they were managing complex ecosystems. When they returned plant and animal wastes to the soil, they were simply creating the conditions that would allow soil organisms to flourish and so nourish their crops.

Where today's industrial farmers are engaged in a relentless battle to subordinate nature and control natural processes, traditional farmers knew this to be pointless. They were content to remain part of the natural process, giving it a nudge here, a prod there, coaxing it in the desired direction. Those who did the job well were repaid with nourishing, nutrient-rich foods. Often they reaped bigger harvests than modern agribusiness, despite its huge arsenal of chemical aids.

The post-industrial view of biology has, until now, failed to register with the policymakers. Organic farming – which embodies the new 'systems' approach – was left to fight it out in the marketplace, where the dice are loaded in favour of large-scale commodity production. Organic food was down-graded into a simple lifestyle choice. All food was nutritious and wholesome, the politicians argued. If a well-off minority wished to pay over the odds for biologically-grown produce, that was their business.

It's a policy that suited both chemical farmers and the supermarkets. In effect it defused any concerted campaign for real foods. Consumers had the choice, therefore govern-ments did not need take to serious action to confront the agribusiness lobby and raise food standards. Now, at last, there's a mood of change in the air.

High-input agriculture has flourished in an environment of generous public support. For decades, western industrial coun-tries have channelled tax revenues into farm subsidies. Now most governments have begun to realize that it's not such a good idea.

In the European Union, the subsidies have already been 'decoupled' from production. This means that farmers are no longer paid by the state for the crops they grow. They're paid instead for the 'public goods' they deliver – a cleaner environ-ment, greater biodiversity, a more beautiful landscape. So long as they keep the land in good condition, they don't have to grow crops at all to receive the cash.

Under Tony Blair's goading, some European countries are pressing for far deeper cuts in public payments to farmers. On the other side of the Atlantic, there are moves for reciprocal cuts in the Unites States. State subsidies have supplied the 'oxygen' that allowed chemical agriculture to grow and pros-per. With the ending of state support there's every chance it will collapse as dramatically as the old Soviet state in the closing years of the twentieth century.

There's far more the politicians could do to hasten change and repair the damage done over decades by their disastrous farm policies. To qualify for the new 'decoupled' support payments, today's farmers have to show they are maintaining their land in good agricultural order. The present rules on 'cross-compliance' set out measures they must take to protect wildlife and avoid physical damage to the soil. What's missing is any requirement to keep soils fertile with a healthy balance of minerals.

It's a simple procedure to analyse soils for important trace elements such as zinc, boron, calcium and selenium, and then make good any deficiencies. A small number of farmers already do it, usually because some health disaster has befallen their crops or their animals. If the government were to make this simple step a condition for collecting support payments, we'd see a dramatic and immediate improvement in the quality of everyday foods.

After decades of neglect, organic farming is now the recipient of new support measures. As a result of recent lobbying, it is becoming clear to the government that an expansion in organic farming may be a way of improving the nation's diet. But it will take years – perhaps decades – to convert Britain to a mainly-organic form of agriculture. Nor is there any guarantee that the foods produced this way will contain the necessary complement of essential minerals.

By introducing the requirement that all farmers balance the soil mineral levels of their soils, the politicians could – at a stroke – improve the health prospects of millions. Under the present rules of 'cross-compliance', food quality ranks below wildlife when it comes to qualifying for the 'single farm payment' scheme.

There are other measures the politicians could quickly make to restore sound husbandry and healthy food. The substitution of green waste compost for chemical fertilizers would produce a near-instant improvement in the health of soils, and with it the health of crops and animals raised on them. Since local authorities were prevented from putting organic wastes into landfill sites in the mid-1990s, small mountains of compost are building up in municipal sites across Britain. It's this compost that should be fertilizing the fields, not the cocktail of chemicals produced by the oil industry.

Intensive livestock farms and nitrate fertilizers – the two are usually linked – cause widespread pollution of watercourses and river estuaries. Under EU legislation farmers in many areas are restricted in the total amount of nitrogen they are allowed to apply per acre. But following intense chemical industry lobbying, the politicians have so far shied away from putting an outright tax on chemical fertilizers.

Yet such a tax would be perfectly justifiable under the 'polluter pays' principle. For a start it could balance the £16 million it costs the water companies each year to remove nitrates from drinking water.[2]

There's an equally strong case for a tax on pesticides, though the government shows every sign of bowing to industry pressure for a voluntary code of practice instead. The water companies spend £120 million a year removing pesticides from drinking water.[3] They don't remove them all, just enough to comply with legal limits. The cost is included in water charges to consumers. This represents a hidden subsidy to those who pollute watercourses and degrade our food.

The Danish government introduced just such a tax in 1996.[4] Weedkillers and fungicides are now taxed at the rate of 34 per cent of the wholesale price, while the rate for the more environmentally-damaging insecticides is more than 50 per cent. Most of the money raised by the tax is returned to farmers in the form of support for more sustainable methods. Along with other measures, the Danish tax has succeeded in cutting the amount of agrochemicals used on farm crops by more than half.

British governments have been far less willing to take on agribusiness interests. It also has to be admitted that in the modern world the freedom of politicians to take decisive action is strictly limited. In all directions they are confronted by powerful political and economic groups – multinational trading companies, the EU, and international regulators such as the World Trade Organization.

There are signs that many in government now recognize the need for radical changes in the way we produce our food. But faced with intense lobbying from special interests, it seems unlikely that they'll act.

The agricultural lobby – dominated over the years by large-scale producers – is likely to oppose the restoration of traditional farming and real food; most family farms have been severely damaged by the shift to commodity production.

Since agriculture came under state control during the Second World War, the economic climate has grown ever more hostile to small family farms, and ever more favourable to large landowners.

Despite it all, Britain still has more than 200,000 small family farms. Disadvantaged by the subsidy system and ignored or opposed by the planners, they have somehow survived. Though their markets have been undermined by commodity producers, they remain more or less intact, awaiting better times. And the better times may be about to arrive.

Large-scale industrial farmers cannot easily convert to good husbandry. Their dependence on agrochemicals and giant machines renders them largely incapable of producing healthy, nutrient-rich foods. By contrast, the small family farm can easily adapt to traditional, biological methods. After all, they're the methods most small farms have been using for centuries.

Opponents may argue that a return to traditional farming will put up the cost of food. There's no disputing that sound farming carries costs that chemical producers manage to evade. Labour costs, for example, are inevitably higher on farms that rely on human skills in place of agrochemicals and giant machines. Against that, there are real savings to be made.

Industrial agriculture imposes hidden costs on the community: the cost of healthcare to combat nutrition-related disease, or the cost of cleaning up polluted watercourses and drinking water supplies. It has been estimated that if we all ate organic foods, the cost of these 'externalities' – which we all pay for in our taxes – would fall by more than one billion pounds annually.[5] The nation as a whole would benefit from a farming system that protected human health and the environment.

> Not long ago I stood on a motorway bridge with the idea of counting the food lorries that passed in an hour. I was on the M5, just north of Weston-super-Mare, at a little after eleven o'clock on a Wednesday morning. After twenty minutes, I'd had enough and went home. By then the total stood at thirty-six, most of them in the livery of the major supermarkets. And I hadn't even counted the unmarked refrigerated trucks that seemed very likely to be carrying food.
>
> Every hour of every day, thousands of food products are hauled across the road system of Britain. Food transport now accounts for a quarter of all the miles driven in the UK by heavy goods vehicles,[6] and it's responsible for almost ten million tonnes of carbon dioxide emissions.

It's worth remembering that in the post-war years, when few families had any money, the entire population – both rich and poor – could afford real food. It's inconceivable that a nation now immeasurably richer could not provide the same for its citizens.

A return to real farming would revitalize rural communities, putting cash in the tills of village shops and more kids into country schools. And the health improvement to the population at large could lead to a national resurgence. It's a revolution Britain can't afford to put off any longer.

There's one group powerful enough to improve food quality almost at will – the supermarkets. With 80 per cent of the grocery trade,[7] supermarkets control what we eat, and, to a large extent, how healthy we are. They don't need to wait for government action. If they chose they could make real food available at a price all their customers could afford. Whether they'll do so without prodding by consumers seems doubtful.

Environmentalists worry about the pollution caused by air-freighting green beans from Kenya or tomatoes from California, but the environmental damage is trivial compared with the trucking of food within Britain. If we were all able to buy food produced within twenty kilometres of where we live, environmental and congestion costs would fall by 90 per cent: or more than £2 billion.[8]

Why should there be all this pollution when there is farmland across the length and breadth of the country? The UK has soils which – when properly looked after – would be among the most fertile and productive in the world. It's soil, not the health service, that is our best assurance of long, healthy lives. Yet we cheerfully abuse it for some spurious notion of convenience offered by the one-stop superstores.

For all their efficiencies, supermarkets as they are currently structured are incapable of delivering truly healthy food. To start with, their centralized buying arrangements mean that even fresh foods must spend hours in warehouses and refrigerated trucks before they even get near the shelves. The supermarkets' cool-chain transport system may well represent a triumph of modern logistics, but it's no substitute for truly fresh food.

Road miles aside, there's much more the major retailers could do to make sure all their customers enjoyed the benefits of real food. They could, for example, insist that their suppliers grew food crops on fertile, well-mineralized soils. An annual soil analysis would quickly highlight fields in which mineral levels were unbalanced, and whose biological activity was in decline. To sell their produce, farmers and growers would have to remedy soil deficiencies. In doing so they might start to question the practices that led to the imbalance in the first place.

From this simple step the retailers would earn much kudos, while suffering no great blow to their margins. They could, if they chose, print on the package a symbol or statement verifying that the product – or its ingredients – had been grown on fertile, well-mineralized soils.

Nor is it beyond the capabilities of fresh produce managers to certify that fruit and vegetable items contained minimal levels of key trace elements. In any food the level of any particular mineral will vary widely according to the variety, growing conditions, climate and so on.

In his experiments in the Forest of Dean, amateur investigator John Reeves (see Chapter 7) devised his own 'mineral score' system to represent the overall content of a range of essential trace elements. What's to stop the supermarkets doing this and guaranteeing that their products contain minimal levels of important trace elements? For example, why not set standards for the micronutrients, magnesium, zinc, chromium and a full range of B vitamins in white bread, instead of simply 'fortifying' with iron, calcium and some vitamins?

They could go very much further to improve the quality of everyday foods. For example, they could insist that at least two-thirds of the milk going into their dairy foods – such as yogurt and cream – is produced by cows grazing fresh, green grass. This would ensure that the products contained decent levels of fat-soluble vitamins, healthy fats – including the protective conjugated linoleic acid – and other important antioxidants. For that matter, what's to stop the retailers setting minimum levels for vitamin and omega-3 fatty acid content?

Supermarkets could equally insist that their beef and lamb was produced largely from grazed grass in summer, and clover-rich hay or silage in winter. So long as the grass is grown on fertile soils, this would result in meats that were truly healthy, at the same time answering many of the criticisms of vegetarians. The same arguments apply to the sourcing of poultry meat and eggs. Those produced largely on fresh pasture would be healthier and more nutritious.

Sadly none of these things is likely to happen without consumer pressure. The reasons are imbedded deep within the culture of modern retailing. Like everything else on the high street, food is principally marketed on price.

'Two for the price of one', shouts the point-of-sale poster. 'Buy one, get one free', or 'Fifty per cent extra free'. Price is the only measure of worth. Foods are seen as no more than material goods, intrinsically no different from cars, freezers and digital cameras. What a contrast in attitude with 'healthy' countries. In those visited by Weston A. Price in the 1930s (see chapter 1), everyone held a deep respect for the land, and for the animals that stocked it. Whenever a new crop was harvested, a fresh batch of butter churned, or an animal killed for its meat, the first response was one of gratitude. The earth had provided the means for life and health. Therefore it was to be honoured.

Modern food retailing allows no such sentiment. In this cut-price culture, food is anonymous. It has no origins and no identity, other than the brand mark of the manufacturer or supermarket.

It may not matter much when it comes to buying a car. It's easy enough to measure quality parameters – how far it goes on a litre of petrol, for example, or the miles travelled between services.

With food it's different. Every fresh item – from an apple to a steak – is infinitely variable in its nutrient content. To begin with, there are the macro nutrients – the proteins, carbohydrates, fats and fibres the food contains. It's not simply the total amounts that matter, it's the quality too. Nutritional value is determined by the form of the proteins, fats and fibre, as well as the amounts present.

At the micro nutrient level, things get even more complicated. The range and proportions of minerals and vitamins have a major bearing on the health-giving quality of foods. Then there are the secondary nutrients or phytonutrients, a bewildering array of up to 10,000 compounds believed to play a part in human health. They include the cancer-preventing glucosinolates found in cabbage, broccoli and Brussels sprouts; carotenoids, the antioxidants found in red or green, leafy vegetables; and the sulphur-containing compounds in onions and garlic that protect against heart disease.

Since the role of many micro-nutrients still has to be established by science, the safest policy would be to ensure their presence by growing foods organically on fertile, well-mineralized soils. Yet supermarkets have little to say on this. They merely ensure that their products are uniform in size and free of blemishes, then sell them as cheaply as possible, always provided there's a good margin in it, of course. It's a policy that is almost bound to depress the nutritional quality of food, and ultimately lead to widespread malnutrition.

The current epidemic of chronic diseases marks the failure of the entire food system, not just of the policymakers. And in that failed system the multiple retailers are major players. By simply offering their customers a choice between chemically-grown 'commodity' foods and 'niche' products such as organic food, the big retailers shirk their responsibility to customers. Fruits and vegetables that are poorly mineralized, meats that are deficient in omega-3 fatty acids – these are not fit for consumption by anyone at any price.

Given the supermarkets' domination of food retailing, many would argue that they have some responsibility for the nutrition of their customers. Currently they choose to sell products like omega-3 enriched milk as high-priced, premium foods. No doubt there will be many more such 'functional foods' as marketing specialists identify new niche markets. But most supermarket shoppers expect such vital nutrients as omega-3s to be present in adequate amounts in ordinary foods – as they would be if those foods were produced by traditional methods.

Perhaps it's time the supermarkets looked again at the nutritional standards of their everyday 'economy' foods. The emergence of nutritionally 'enhanced' foods suggests that the economy equivalent is, in some aspects at least, nutritionally depleted. The big retailers could be seen as being more concerned to maximize their market revenue than with the health and well-being of their customers.

In the end it must be consumers themselves who bring about change. By the way we vote we can make good farming and healthy food a real political issue. And through our dialogue with shops and supermarkets, we can begin to make the nutritional value of foods a retail priority.

As Patrick Holden points out (see page 187), given the supermarkets' sensitivity to consumer trends, the transformation could come about very quickly. One of the chief drivers in modern retailing is the fear of losing market share. So obsessed are the major players to stay ahead in the race, they watch tirelessly for new and changing customer attitudes. Complaints and suggestions are usually monitored at board level. Anything that looks like a genuine shift in consumer tastes – and this could include a growing interest in 'real food' – is quickly picked up and acted upon.

In the world of multiple retailing, it needn't take a popular mass movement to bring about substantial change. A demand for better food from even a small percentage of a supermarket's customers could spark a small revolution at store level.

A few simple questions to in-store staff could become a powerful force for change (see also Chapter 13). For example, when buying beef it's worth asking the butcher or fresh-produce manager whether the cut on offer is from a mostly grass-fed animal. What you need to find out is how much of its life did the animal spend grazing grass, and for those periods it was inside, what it was fed on. Small amounts of grain are acceptable so long as the diet was made up principally of fibrous feeds, such as hay and grass clover silage.

What you're after is basic information about how the animal is produced. Good butchers – either in a supermarket or in the high street – should be able to supply the information. If they can't, make sure you challenge them again next time you're in the store. Without a basic knowledge of the production process it's impossible to make a sound judgement about which foods are healthy and which are best left alone.

As for meat, so for milk and dairy products. It's well worth asking the supermarket how big a proportion is from cows grazing fresh grass. The question is quite likely to bring a blank stare, but the point will have been made. Since New Zealand butter is produced from grazed grass, it might be worth asking whether there's a British brand that can make the same claim. There probably won't be, but again the point will have been made.

For butter, cheese and milk from exclusively grass- and forage-fed cows, the most likely source is a farmers' market or the Internet. Even so, it's worth asking at the supermarket. When the multiples start getting asked for the real stuff, it won't be long before they talk to their suppliers about sourcing it. Until that day the best policy is to choose organic. This will at least ensure that a large part of the animals' diet is in the form of grass and forage crops.

When it comes to bread, biscuits and cakes made from properly-mineralized wheat, there's a battle ahead. Today's wheat growers are in the business not of producing food but turning out a raw material for manufacturing industry. When they speak of quality it's not the nutrient content of the grains they're talking about, but how closely its physical characteristics meet the requirements of industrial millers and plant bakers.

Since the milling process itself removes a sizeable proportion of the nutrients, why worry about the levels in the grain? Nutrient content can be left to the bakers. They will 'fortify' the flour with whatever vitamins and minerals the law tells them to, or with those they think will give them a marketing edge. In practice that means just a handful of nutrients to replace the dozens that are lost or depleted during milling and baking.

The result is every time we pick up a sandwich at the supermarket's 'local' convenience store, we're buying a product whose nutritional value is doubtful.

At the moment the only way to get a half-decent sandwich is to find an outlet that uses only organically-grown ingredients. Even then there's no guarantee that the flour will have contained decent levels of minerals and vitamins. The emergence of the truly healthy sandwich will have to await a change in the mindset of arable farmers. For that to happen, retailers – particularly the supermarkets – will need to take more responsibility for the ingredients that go into the processed and manufactured products they sell.

It's we as consumers who will bring about the food renaissance. By insisting on 'real food' we could transform the health of the nation. Even the notorious fast-foods we have become so attached to – the pizzas and the burgers on sale in every high street – could be made to deliver more of the nutrients that protect health, rather than undermining it.

13
Delving Deeper

Imagine a company whose new products are inferior to what has gone before – a computer firm whose latest model is slower than the old one, a car company whose new model has a top speed of 30mph and needs a starting handle to get it going. The odds are that sales would be slow.

Yet in the world of everyday foods this is the norm. Many of the familiar staple foods that fill the shelves of modern supermarkets are nutritionally inferior to those our parents and grandparents ate. Unlike car and computer manufacturers, food producers can get away with this 'dumbing down' of their products, simply because science has yet to find a way of analysing the total nutrient content.

The big retailers stock their stores with foods that look fresh and unblemished, but in terms of their power to promote health and fitness they are mostly second-rate. There are still good, healthy foods out there, mostly in small quantities that are easily lost in the jungle that is the modern food system. They're known only to those intrepid 'foodies' who take the trouble to seek them out.

For most of us who visit supermarkets and want fast, hassle-free shopping, it's the second-rate we get. In modern food retailing this is the 'default' position. Finding nutrient-rich foods that will promote the health of our families takes time, and until now few of us have been prepared to go to the trouble.

Yet is it really such a commitment? It needn't take any more effort than arranging the annual family holiday, and the pay-off in good health will be a lot longer lasting. There's also the satisfaction of knowing that the more of us who go to the trouble of seeking out real food, the faster it will become available in the mainstream food outlets.

In the search for real food, there's one vital step that will help to ensure success. Wherever possible, choose food with an 'identity'. For fresh foods this means those that come from identified farms, with the full farm details supplied by the retailer or printed on the accompanying packaging.

Knowing the origins of a food changes the relationship between producer and consumer. If you know where a food comes from, you can act on your experience of it. If you've been disappointed, you can complain. If you're worried about some aspect of the production process, you can call the farmer and discuss it. If you're still unhappy, you can walk away and buy elsewhere.

Of course you may be perfectly happy with a food and feel no need to contact the producer. The mere fact that you have the farm details will ensure the farmer works hard to bring you a good product that you'll want to go on buying in the future.

One of the most damaging consequences of the political management of agriculture is that it placed bureaucracy be-tween farmers and their customers. Farmers quickly lost interest in what happened to their products once they'd dis-appeared through the farm gate. All they had to do was ensure their products met the minimum standards of the Ministry grader or the official EU intervention store (where surplus production was held). After that, they could forget them. Their products would be lost in the great sea of commodity foods everyone was obliged to eat.

For the consumer there was no one to complain to, no one to listen to concerns about aspects of the production process. There were officials to take care of all that. As far as food was concerned this was very much a 'Big Brother state', where the interests of consumers were looked after by Whitehall and by Brussels.

It was an arrangement that managed to swamp farmers beneath a torrent of form-filling and bureaucracy while giving them little incentive to improve the nutritional quality of their products. Britain was still subjected to regular food scares, from BSE and its human equivalent – new-variant CJD – to bovine TB. Yet ordinary citizens were denied any say in the way their basic foods were produced.

Today the gateway to farming and food production is guarded not by the Ministry bureaucrat but by the supermarkets and the big food companies. With the politicians now largely discredited as protectors of the food supply, the retailers and the food industry are trying hard to win the nation's trust. They, too, have an interest in keeping their suppliers anonymous.

In order to minimize procurement costs, they want the freedom to switch easily from one supplier to another. In this way producers can be played off against each other, so driving down prices. By identifying the producer of a particular food they risk turning it into a brand with its own loyal following, a development that would severely limit their control and, ultimately, their profitability.

I know a dairy farmer who has for many years packaged his premium-quality milk in his own distinctive cartons and supplied one of the major supermarket chains. Recently, the supermarket decided it wanted to 'rationalize' the supply of quality milk, selling the output of fewer producers under its own label. My friend was told his milk was no longer required and his cartons were removed from the chill cabinet.

Within days the volume of customer complaints had swelled to an avalanche. They demanded that the familiar cartons be returned to the shelves. They had grown to love the delicious, creamy milk produced from clover-filled pastures, and they were determined to get it back. In the face of such clear customer demand, the supermarket was forced to reinstate the product.

Knowing the origins of foods puts power back in the hands of consumers and keeps producers on their mettle. Increasingly the best fresh foods carry the name of the producer. Under the weight of public pressure, even the supermarkets are adorning their stores – and their packaging – with photos of smiling farmers standing in front of grazing cows or a bunch of outdoor pigs. At the moment they're largely restricted to the 'premium' end of the market, particularly organic foods, but in other retail outlets, such as farm shops and farmers' markets, the farmer ID has become standard.

WHY NOT ASK QUESTIONS?

Simply knowing the origin of a food should in itself give you confidence in it. The farmer has been brave enough to take responsibility for the product, so there's every likelihood it will have been produced with integrity. Even so, there's a lot to be gained by entering into a fuller dialogue. By asking the right questions, there's much to be learned about the production process, which is ultimately the best guide to the nutritional value of a food.

Having noted the grower's name and address, look up the website – if there is one – and see how much information it provides. If there's more you need to ask, phone the farmer at a convenient time. Evenings are best. Even better, make an appointment to visit the farm. Farmers are busy, hard-working people, but they might be willing to show off their workplace to visitors. Alternatively, talk to them at markets.

Having made contact with the farmer, it's worth giving some thought to the information you want. It will help you choose the tastiest, healthiest food available.

Nutritious milk and healthy dairy products

The natural food for dairy cows is green vegetation, especially the fast-growing grasses of spring and early summer. The best milk comes from cows grazing on fertile pastures containing plenty of clover and herbs. In many parts of lowland Britain, cattle will happily live outdoors all year without ill effects, but to save their pastures from being damaged during wet weather, most farmers prefer to bring their cattle inside for the winter months.

Choose a farm where the cows are out on pasture for at least six months of the year, though eight or nine is better. Many traditional farmers grazed their cows on other forage crops, such as cereals, kale and turnip greens, during the winter months. These are natural foods for ruminant animals, and helped to produce high-quality milk at a difficult time of the year. Few herds are managed this way today, but a little consumer persuasion could bring about a rapid change.

The farmer should be using little or no chemical fertilizer. A good indicator of a healthy, fertile soil is an abundance of clover in the 'sward', together with a number of different grasses and herbs.

Find out what the cows are fed on when they're brought inside. After fresh, growing plants, the best foods are hay or silage made from the same clover and herb-rich grasslands. These bulky foods should make up the larger part of the ration. Ideally, they should be supplemented with a home-mixed ration containing oats, linseed and beans.

Steer clear of herds where soya meal is fed in winter. Unfortunately, this will rule out most of Britain's large commercial dairy herds, but soya as a feed is unhealthy for ruminant animals, and too little research has been done on its effects on the protein in milk.[1] Also avoid herds feeding on large amounts of starchy foods, whether in the form of cereals or bakery waste.

Small herds are best, anything up to around seventy cows. There are still plenty of them about. As for breed, I would choose a farm with one of the traditional British dairy cows – the Ayrshire, the Shorthorn, the Guernsey, the Jersey or the traditional British Friesian. Most modern Holsteins have been turned into walking 'milk factories', to the detriment of milk quality.

Edward Howell, who had a lifelong interest in the health benefits of enzymes, particularly those in unpasteurized milk, wrote in his book *Enzyme Nutrition*: 'The interests of mass production have led to the selection of cows with abnormally large udders. The so-called "scrub cows" of former times, with their small udders and less milk secretion, had less strain on their metabolism and could produce milk of higher health value.'[2]

Best beef

The chief requirement for healthy beef is the same as for milk – a fertile pasture with plentiful clover and herbs. The use of chemical fertilizers should be low or non-existent. A good way to check is to find out how species-rich the pastures are. If they contain a range of different grasses – plus clovers and herbs – it's a fair bet there aren't too many chemical fertilizers going on.

Choose one of the older British breeds, such as the traditional Hereford (the uncommon original type, very different from the larger, modern Hereford) the Devon or 'Red Ruby', the Welsh Black, the Lincoln Red, the Beef Shorthorn, the Galloway, the Aberdeen Angus or the Sussex. Many of these breeds have been 'improved' in recent years by crossing with an outside breed to meet modern requirements.[3] This can result in some valuable traits of the original animal being lost, so it's worth making sure the farmer keeps the traditional type.

Thanks to the work of the Rare Breeds Survival Trust, it's possible to go further. There is a wide range of even rarer breeds, each with its own distinctive qualities. They include the White Park – the oldest recorded beef breed in Britain – and the Dexter. These were livestock bred to thrive on grass. Their beef is more likely to be rich in essential omega-3 fats, conjugated linoleic acid and vitamins than the modernized type. It's not difficult to find 'rare breed beef'. Log on to the RBST website to find your nearest accredited rare-breeds butcher.[4]

A word of warning if you're asking about beef breeds in your local supermarket. Some supermarket schemes claiming to support traditional beef breeds require only that the farmer uses a bull of that breed. The beef may well come from a cross-bred animal in which the benefits will be considerably diluted.

As mentioned before, for the healthiest beef, the animal needs to have spent much of its life grazing on pasture. During the winter months 'yarding' on clover-rich hay or silage is fine, as are a limited amount of cereals during the finishing period. The cereals should have been home-grown on a fertile soil and not be of the chemically-grown industrial variety.

Raising proper, grass-fed beef is necessarily a slow process. Don't expect to buy traditional-breed beef younger than twenty-eight months of age. After slaughter it should have been properly hung for two to three weeks.

You'd think all this care would make real beef expensive, but it shouldn't be. I know a farmer who raises pedigree Devon cattle in fields so full of summer flowers they look like Alpine meadows. His cattle are magnificent, and he makes good money for those he sells as breeding stock. The rest are slaughtered when ready and put into the commercial food chain, where they're sold for the same price as cattle kept in sheds and fed a ton of cereals.

It's worth going to some trouble to find farmers like that. In nutritional terms, their beef is priceless.

Eggs and poultry

You're unlikely to find the best eggs in a supermarket. The healthiest eggs come from hens running on fresh, green forage every day. This means they must be kept in portable houses that can be moved daily to a new pasture paddock.

Keeping the birds on fresh grass, while protecting them from predators like foxes and stoats, is a demanding and skilful undertaking. The big producers prefer to keep their massive flocks in sheds and cages, manipulating some ingredient in their industrial rations to produce some desirable characteristic in the egg, such as the level of omega-3 fats. Even free-range producers find it hard to organize the move to fresh new pasture every day.

Yet this is crucial if you want truly healthy eggs and

chickens. To stay healthy, hens need fresh air, sunlight, earth, exercise and about 60 gm of fresh, green food every day.[5] Old, worn pastures that have been pecked and scratched over for the past two weeks won't do. To produce healthy eggs and meat they must get their ration of fresh, clover-rich pasture daily.

The green food will provide B vitamins and carotenes, some of which the chicken will turn into vitamin A.[6] Omega-3 fatty acids in the forage will end up in the fat, and exposure to sunlight ensures that the fat will also contain vitamin D. The more yellow the fat, the more nutritious the chicken. The same applies to eggs. The characteristic deep orange-coloured yolk from pasture-fed chicken is a sign that the egg is rich in vitamins and essential fats.

In the United States pasture poultry production – based on the portable shed or 'Eggmobile' – is growing in popularity. To get over the predator threat, some producers have 'bonded' dogs with hens, training them to mount guard over the birds.

In the UK, this kind of transient poultry production is more likely to be practised by smallholders and 'good-lifers' than mainstream farmers. Farmers' markets and WI Country Markets are more promising places to search them out than your average neighbourhood supermarket.

Sweet-tasting lamb

Lamb ought to be the healthiest of meats. Most lambs are raised on pasture, so their meat should be rich in essential fatty acids, fat-soluble vitamins and minerals. The ones to be wary of are those from early-lambing flocks that are finished quickly for marketing in February and March. Farmers rely on cereal-feeding to meet this high-priced early market. It's well worth treating lamb as a seasonal food and waiting till early summer for the first ones to fatten on grass.

The other practice that spoils lamb as a universally healthy food is the widespread use of nitrogen fertilizer. Sheep farmers are as attached to heavily-fertilized grass monocultures as other livestock producers. Lamb coming off this sort of 'forced' grass are unlikely to be so well mineralized as those of species-rich pastures with plenty of clover and deep-rooting herbs. Slow-growing lambs from mountain pastures or salt marshes can be among the tastiest and most nutritious.

It's worth seeking out a traditional breed, too. There are dozens of British sheep breeds, reflecting a time when animals were adapted to local conditions. Today many are in decline or are out-and-out rarities. Efficiency-minded farmers have standardized on the Mule ewe – usually a cross between a Blue-faced Leicester and a Blackface or Swaledale – chosen for its prolificacy and mothering qualities, and a Texel ram. However, for taste and nutritional quality, it's worth asking the butcher – or searching the farmers' market – for one of the traditional breeds, such as the Shropshire, Southdown, Portland, Llanwenog, Cheviot or Hampshire.

For an unrivalled taste experience – and a healthy one – try out some of the rarer, primitive breeds, such as the Soay, the Castlemilk Moorit, the Hebridean, the Manx Shetland and the North Ronaldsay. These can be described as Neolithic sheep in the sense that they are direct descendants. As a result, they are generally long-living and healthy, and – unlike most modern commercial breeds – cannot be induced to grow too quickly. This ensures that their meat is flavoursome and healthy.

Alternatively, it's worth trying some of the other rare breeds, such as the White Face Dartmoor, the Norfolk Horn, the White Faced Woodland, the Portland, the Southdown and the Ryeland. The list seems endless – a real gourmet's delight. It's one of the ironies of farming that some of the wildest, most wind-swept pastures can produce the sweetest-tasting, healthiest sheep-meat around.

Bread

Finding good bread is likely to be one of the toughest tasks in the hunt for real food. Wherever you look, be sure to ask questions about the flour used. It's important to choose bread from wheat – or other grains – grown on fertile, well-mineralized soil. At the very least they should have been grown to organic standards, so they are free of pesticide residues. Ideally the land should also have been subjected to regular trace element analysis.

It's equally important that the grain is handled properly in preparation for baking. The whole grain should have been traditionally stone ground – or milled with slow-speed steel hammer mills – to preserve the valuable minerals, vitamins and essential fats.

Wheat, like other grains, contains an organic acid called phytic acid in the outer layer or bran. Untreated phytic acid can combine with calcium, magnesium, copper, iron and zinc in the intestinal tract, blocking the absorption of these essential minerals.[7] As a result, a diet high in unfermented whole grains can lead to serious mineral deficiencies and even bone loss. That's why the modern practice of eating large amounts of unprocessed bran to improve bowel action can also lead to adverse side effects, such as irritable bowel syndrome. Traditional societies almost always soak or ferment whole grains before they use them. Soaking allows enzymes and beneficial micro-organisms to break down and neutralize phytic acid. The simple practice of soaking cracked or rolled cereal grains overnight greatly improves their nutritional qualities.

Unless you're prepared to bake your own bread, look for organic sourdough and sprouted breads at the farmers' market or wholefood shop. Sourdough leavening is the traditional method of bread-making, using wild yeast in place of modern fast yeasts. It's a slower process, which allows the grains to be 'pre-digested', so that the nutrients can be more easily absorbed and metabolized.

Sprouting means allowing the grains to start germinating, a process that increases enzyme activity and inactivates substances called enzyme inhibitors, which would otherwise hinder digestion. American research has shown that sprouting increases the total nutrient density of foods.[8] Whole wheat from sprouted grains was found to contain up to three times more vitamin C, folic acid, riboflavin (vitamin B2), niacin (vitamin B3), pantothenic acid (vitamin B5), biotin and thiamine (vitamin B1), than non-sprouted whole wheat.

WHERE CAN YOU FIND REAL FOOD?

If you're a regular supermarket shopper, it's worth starting the search there. Real food isn't unheard of in the giant super-stores, it's simply that the cut-price culture of modern grocery retailing is more likely to drive down food quality than force it up, even for premium foods such as organic.

While the organic label will certainly steer you away from foods that are laden with pesticide residues, it won't be a foolproof guide to foods that are nutrient-rich. For example, a pack of organic apples are not guaranteed to be well-endowed with trace minerals. You'll need a Brix refractometer (see Chapter 2) or a set of well-educated taste buds to find that out.

An organic label on the milk carton will guarantee that at least 60 per cent of the cows' diet was in the form of fibrous fodder, fresh or dried. What it won't tell you is how much of the diet was in the form of fresh, grazed pasture, the food that secures the highest content of health-giving vitamins and omega-3 fats in the milk. While supermarket organic milk may meet the minimum standards, it won't compare in its health-giving properties with the milk of spring-calving cows grazed on fresh pastures until December.

The chances are that close scrutiny of most supermarket foods will point up serious deficiencies for those in search of truly healthy foods. That's when it's time to start looking elsewhere.

Farmers' markets

Farmers' markets have produced something of a food retailing revolution over the past few years. The first opened in Bath in 1997, and there are now around 500 operating across the UK. They are used by almost one-third of the population.[9]

The basic principles of farmers' markets are that the food on sale must have been produced locally – often within fifty miles – and that the person selling the produce must have been involved in its production. These rules make farmers' markets an ideal place to meet farmers and quiz them about aspects of the production process. There's a chance to ask beef producers how long their animals spend grazing and how many plant species there are in the pastures. On stalls selling vegetables, there's the opportunity to find out from growers how they ensure the soil is fertile and rich in available minerals.

Farmers' markets vary widely in the range of produce they offer and their general dynamism as retail operations. My own local market – in a Somerset seaside town – is a fairly dismal affair. It's held in a church hall well away from the main shopping area, and while the foods on offer are generally good, the range of produce is disappointing.

A survey of farmers' markets in the south-west region showed that shoppers could expect to pay at least one-third less at farmers' markets than for items of a similar quality bought at supermarkets.[10]

Farm shops

These are another good place to meet farmers and find out more about their production methods. As the name implies, farm shops are generally attached to farms with at least some of the produce being grown and raised on the home fields. Many shops stock meat, eggs, fruit and vegetables, plus a range of local and regional products, such as jams and chutneys.

There are now more than 3,000 farm shops in the UK, excluding farms that simply sell the odd item from the 'farm gate'. Since most of the foods are produced 'at home' or on an identified local farm, there's a chance to make contact with the producer and discover more about how the foods are grown.

In addition to the traditional farm shop, there's now a new breed of town centre store, a sort of hybrid between farm shops and farmers' markets. The Goods Shed in Canterbury describes itself as Britain's first daily farmers' market and food hall. It was set up by a group of Kent farmers, growers, fishermen and cider producers, who wanted a permanent outlet for their products. They operate it along cooperative lines, employing paid staff to run the stalls.

Though farmers or their staff aren't actually on site at this type of shop, staff are well-informed about the produce they sell. For detailed explanations of the production process, they may need to refer back to producers.

Box schemes

Box schemes represent growing forms of direct marketing in the UK. Originally developed by organic vegetable growers who wanted to short-circuit the lengthy food supply chain, they have now been taken up by producers of fruit, dairy produce, meat and wine. They have become a principal means of getting food direct from farmers to consumers.

There are now around 400 box schemes operating in Britain, three-quarters of them supplying organic produce. They provide a means for entering into a long-term relationship with food producers. Box scheme customers are encouraged to provide feedback to the producer about what they've enjoyed and what they don't like. There's no reason why the dialogue shouldn't be expanded to include the production methods used and how they could be improved.

When a vegetable supplied in a box scheme lacks flavour, for example, there's a mechanism for alerting the producer and pressing for improvements. If you have a Brix refractometer (see Chapter 2), back up your complaint with the readings. Suggest that the farmer has the soil analysed, and where it is deficient takes steps to remedy it.

Box schemes have many benefits for farmers and growers. They offer a secure market, stable prices and a regular income. That's why few producers running them will want to lose customers. There's every incentive to keep consumers happy by growing better foods.

The Internet

A UK web search for 'grass-fed' produced around 10,000 hits. Many were on the science of pasture feeding and its effects on omega-3 levels in the meat. There were also a fair number of sites offering grass-fed beef for home delivery. One of the best sites – a resource called Seeds of Health – featured a number of articles on the health benefits of pasture-fed beef and milk, together with a list of suppliers.[11]

The Internet has become an important route for sourcing real food. Farm websites generally give a brief outline of their production process. In the case of beef they'll normally identify the breeds used and whether they're mainly grass-fed. When in doubt, there's always a phone number and an e-mail address for further contact.

Run a search for 'organic, food, direct' in the UK and you'll come up with more than a million hits. Type in 'natural, food, direct' and you'll come up with nearly five million pages. Direct sales of food are booming. In 2004, direct organic food sales grew by 16 per cent to £108 million, while food sales through supermarkets fell.[12]

The Internet is proving a powerful force in the struggle for healthier foods. It is enabling health-conscious consumers to make direct contact with producers without having to go through the tangle of processors, distributors and large retailers that make up the modern food system. It gives consumers a fast, direct means of making their requirements clear to farmers, and it gives farmers a clear incentive to respond. The Net looks capable of making real food available to everyone.

Community-supported agriculture (CSA)

Community most demanding – and perhaps the most rewarding – way of securing healthy food for the family. Basically, a group of consumers get together and contract a local farm to produce the kind of foods they want using the methods they're happy with. Sometimes it's simply a matter of guaranteeing farmers an agreed annual income in return for producing the right kinds of food. In a few cases, community groups have taken on farms themselves, simply engaging local farmers to manage the holdings on a paid basis.

In all its forms, CSA demands a big commitment from consumers. To a greater or lesser extent they are taking on responsibility for the production and delivery of healthy food. In Stroud in Gloucestershire, one hundred families make a fixed monthly payment to Stroud Community Agriculture. The money pays for the services of three part-time farmers, the rent on 23 acres of land, and everything else needed to produce vegetables, beef and pork from healthy, fertile soils.

The scheme aims to share the risks and rewards of good farming between farmers and consumers. Consumers make a commitment to support the farm and provide a fair income for the farmers. This means the farmers then have the security to develop the health and fertility of the land. The produce is shared among the supporting members. When there's a surplus it's sold locally, though with a waiting list of families keen to join, there are few surpluses these days.

Notes

Chapter 1

1. E. Walter Russell, *Soil Conditions and Plant Growth*, 9th edn, Longman, 1961, p. 183. Russell quotes figures from the long-running Broadbalk experiment at Rothamsted experimental station in Hertfordshire. A plot fertilized with organic manure contained one million earthworms to the acre, weighing 200kg. Plots receiving heavy dressings of chemical fertilizer contained fewer than half the number of worms, weighing between 22kg and 45kg an acre.
2. Marc David, *Nourishing Wisdom: A Mind–Body Approach to Nutrition and Well-being*, cited in Sally Fallon, *Nourishing Traditions*, revised 2nd Edn, New Trends Publishing, 2001, p. 538.
3. Gene Logsdon, 'All Flesh is Grass', in Norman Wirzba (ed.), *The Essential Agrarian Reader*, University Press of Kentucky, 2003, pp. 154–70.

Chapter 2

1. Weston A. Price, *Nutrition and Physical Degeneration*, 6th edn, Price-Pottenger Nutrition Foundation, 2004.
2. Price began his gigantic study on root canal infections in 1900. In 1915, the National Dental Association – later to become the American Dental Association – appointed him as their first research director. Leading a research team of sixty, he published his findings in 1923. They appeared in two volumes – *Dental*

Infections Oral and Systemic and *Dental Infections and Degenerative Diseases*. The first volume is currently published by the Price-Pottenger Nutrition Foundation.

3. Rex Harrill, *Using a Refractometer to Test the Quality of Fruits and Vegetables*, Pineknoll Publishing, 1994.
4. Sally Fallon, *Nourishing Trends*, revised 2nd edn, New Trends Publishing, 2001, pp. 40-45.
5. Peter Crawford, *The Living Isles – A Natural History of Britain and Ireland*, BBC, 1985, p. 64.
6. Douglas Palmer (ed.), *The Illustrated Encyclopedia of Dinosaurs and Prehistoric Animals*, Marshall Publishing, 1988, p. 279.
7. An unusually large race of red deer still occupy forest land in the west of Ireland. Known as the giant red stags of Connemara, they were re-introduced by an estate owner, following the shooting of the original deer during the famines of the 1840s. The introduced stags have astonished deer experts by growing to an immense size. One of the reasons for their size – and the dimensions of their antlers – is thought to be the underlying limestone, which supplies large amounts of calcium via the vegetation. Duff Hart-Davis, 'The Antler Heroes', *Daily Telegraph*, 14 May 2005.

Chapter 3

1. Patrick Holford, *New Optimum Nutrition Bible*, Piatkus, 2004, p. 269.
2. Surgeon Captain T.L. Cleave, *The Saccharine Disease*, John Wright, 1974.
3. Dr Walter Yellowlees, 'Ill Fares the Land', in *Soil, Food and Health*, Wholefood Trust, 1989, pp. 15–42.
4. Originally published by Faber, the book was later republished by the McCarrison Society. R. McCarrison, *Nutrition and Health*, Westbury Press, 1982.
5. Sulphonamide – a drug developed in the 1930s from the red dye prontosil – was found to have powerful antimicrobial properties, particularly against streptococcus bacteria. The discovery was made in 1933 by the German chemist Gerhard Domagk, director of research for the company Bayer. Using derivatives of sulphonamide, chemists went on to develop treatments for hypertension, diabetes, heart failure, glaucoma, thyrotoxicosis, malaria and leprosy. See James Le Fanu, *The Rise and Fall of Modern Medicine*, Little Brown, 1999, pp. 210–15.
6. James Le Fanu, op. cit., p. 210.
7. *Cancer Trends in England and Wales 1950–1999*, Office for National Statistics, 2005.

8. *Coronary Heart Disease Statistics 2005*, British Heart Foundation, June 2005.
9. L.J. Melton, E.J. Atkinson, M.K. O'Connor, et al., 'Bone Density and Fracture Risk in Men', *Journal of Bone Mineral Research*, 1998, Vol. 13, p. 1915; L.J. Melton, E.A. Chrischilles, C. Cooper, et al., 'Perspective: How Many Women Have Osteoporosis?', *Journal of Bone Mineral Research* 1992, Vol. 7, p. 1005.
10. *Compendium of Health Statistics*, 16th edn, 2004–5, Office for Health Economics.
11. Raymond Steen, 'Beef: A Naturally Healthy Product', *Beef Farmer* Spring 2000, pp. 17–18.

Chapter 4

1. David Thomas, 'A Study on the Mineral Depletion of the Foods Available to Us as a Nation Over the Period 1940 to 1991', *Nutrition and Health* 2003, Vol. 17, pp. 85–115.
2. Tom Stockdale, 'Coronary Heart Disease: A New Perspective', *Nutrition and Health*, 2004, Vol. 18, pp. 73–75. Stockdale argues that a marginal deficiency in selenium over many years causes coronary heart disease. He links the continuing high UK incidence of the disease to the switch from Canadian hard wheats to European wheats by this country's flour millers. From the late nineteenth century, selenium-rich Canadian wheat used to produce the standard white loaf that protected UK consumers from deficiency diseases. But since the ending of Canadian wheat imports in the 1980s, a considerable proportion of the UK population has suffered from one or more symptoms of selenium deficiency, while those who were already marginally deficient are now severely affected. This last group are subject to a range of conditions including obesity, late onset diabetes, ADHD and depression.
3. M.P. Rayman, 'The Argument for Increasing Selenium Intake', *Proceedings of the Nutrition Society* Vol. 61, pp. 203–15.
4. Colin Tudge, *So Shall We Reap*, Allen Lane, 2003, pp. 108–9.
5. Nigel Hawkes, 'Vitamin Boost for Young Criminals Cuts Offence Rate', *The Times*, 26 June 2002.
6. Jane Seymour, 'Hungry For a New Revolution', *New Scientist* 30 March 1996.
7. *Diet, Nutrition and the Prevention of Chronic Diseases*, Report of the Joint WHO/FAO Expert Consultation, April 2002.
8. Maynard Murray, *Sea Energy Agriculture*, revised 2nd edn, Acres USA, 2003, p. 31.

9. André Voisin, *Soil, Grass and Cancer*, Acres USA, 1999, p. 1.
10. Max B. Lurie, *Resistance to Tuberculosis: Experimental Studies in Native and Acquired Defensive Mechanisms*, Harvard University Press, 1964.
11. Helen Fullerton, *Bovine Tuberculosis: A Nutritional Solution*, Farming and Livestock Concern UK, 2002.

Chapter 5

1. Pesticide Residues Committee, *Annual Report 2003*. http://www.pesticides.gov.uk
2. Caroline Cox, 'Herbicide Factsheet: Glyphosate (Roundup)', *Journal of Pesticide Reform* 1998, Vol. 18, No. 3, pp. 3–17.
3. W.S. Pease et al., 'Preventing Pesticide-Related Illness in California Agriculture: Strategies and Priorities', *Environmental Health Policy Program Report*, Berkeley, CA, 1993, University of California School of Public Health Policy Seminar.
4. California Environmental Protection Agency, Department of Pesticide Regulation, Case Reports Received by the California Pesticide Illness Surveillance Program in Which Health Effects were Attributed to Glyphosate, 1998, Unpublished Report, Sacramento, CA, cited in Caroline Cox, op. cit.
5. California Environmental Protection Agency, Department of Pesticide Regulation, Worker Health and Safety Branch. Case Reports Received by the California Pesticide Illness Surveillance Program, in which health effects were attributed to exposure to malathion, alone or in combination, 2003, Unpublished Database, cited in Caroline Cox, 'Insecticide Factsheet: Malathion', *Journal of Pesticide Reform* 2003, Vol. 23, No. 4, pp. 10–15.
6. Ibid.
7. G. Cabello et al., 'A Rat Mammary Tumor Model Induced by the Organophosphorous Pesticides Parathion and Malathion, Possibly Through Acetylcholinesterase Inhibition', *Environmental Health Perspectives* 2001, 109, pp. 471–9.
8. Vyvyan Howard, 'Synergistic Effects of Chemical Mixtures – Can We Rely on Traditional Toxicology?', *The Ecologist* 1997, Vol. 27, No. 5, pp. 192–95.
9. Ontario College of Family Physicians, Review of Research on the Effects of Pesticides on Human Health, 2004. http://www.ocfp.on.ca
10. Albert Howard, 'Soil Fertility', in H. J. Massingham (ed.), *England and the Farmer*, Batsford, 1941.
11. Alison Burrell et al., *Statistical Handbook of UK Agriculture*,

Macmillan, 1984, p. 98. Department of Environment, Food and Rural Affairs, '2005 Harvest: Provisional Estimates of Cereal Production United Kingdom', 13 October 2005.

12. Vandana Shiva, 'Globalization and the War Against Farmers and the Land', in Norman Wirzba (ed.), *The Essential Agrarian Reader*, Kentucky University Press, 2003.

13. The comparison was made in a conversation between Mr Furuno and a group of mono-crop rice growers from Texas. The conversation is reported by North Dakota organic farmer Frederick Kirschenmann, who is also director of the Leopold Center at Iowa State University. See: Frederick Kirschenmann, 'The Current State of Agriculture: Does It Have a Future?' in Norman Wirzba, op. cit.

14. Marc Bonfils studied and travelled in Africa, researching traditional tribal agriculture in his hunt for methods that worked with nature rather than against it. He was greatly influenced by the work of Japanese farmer Masanobu Fukuoka, and has adapted many of his natural farming methods to European conditions. See Mark Moodie, *The Harmonious Wheatsmith*, available from eco-logic books, 19 Maple Grove, Bath, BA2 3AF. http://www.eco-logicbooks.com. Bonfils himself authored a number of works, including *Culture Du Blé d'Hiver,* available from Las Encantadas, B. P. 217, F-11300, Limoux, France.

15. William C. Edgar, *The Story of a Grain of Wheat*, London: George Newnes, 1902, pp. 13–14.

16. Sally Fallon, *Nourishing Traditions*, New Trends Publishing, 1999, p. 24.

17. Gene Logsdon, 'All Flesh is Grass' in Norman Wirzba (ed.), *The Essential Agrarian Reader*, University Press of Kentucky, 2003, pp. 154–70.

Chapter 6

1. Newman Turner, *Fertility Farming*, Faber and Faber, 1951, pp. 67–8.

2. Robert H. Elliot, *The Clifton Park System of Farming*, Faber and Faber, 1898, p. 139.

3. J.A. Scimeca et al., 'Conjugated Linoleic Acid: A Powerful Anti-Carcinogen From Animal Fat Sources', *Cancer* 1994, Vol. 74 (3 suppl.), pp. 1050–4.

4. T.R. Dhiman et al., 'Conjugated Linoleic Acid Content of Milk From Cows Fed Different Diets', *Journal of Dairy Science* 1999, Vol. 82 (10), 2146–56.

5. Richard Manning, *Grassland: The History, Biology, Politics, and Promise of the American Prairie*, Penguin Books USA, 1995, p. 127.

6. S.K. Duckett et al., 'Effects of Time of Feed on Beef Nutrient Composition', *Journal of Animal Science*, 1993, Vol. 71 (8), pp. 2079–88.

7. T.A. Dolecek et al., 'Dietary Polyunsaturated Fatty Acids and Mortality in the Multiple Risk Factor Intervention Trial (MRFIT)', *World Review of Nutrition and Dietetics* 1991, Vol. 66, pp. 205–16.

8. English Beef and Lamb Executive, 'Latest Finisher Costings Give CAP Reform Hope', Briefing Note No. 04/14, September 2004.

9. Artemis P. Simopoulos, 'n-3 Fatty Acids and Human Health: Defining Strategies for Public Policy', *Lipids* 2001, Vol. 36, Supplement, pp. S83–89.

10. Associate Parliamentary Food and Health Forum, Evidence Given to Joint Meeting on Diet and Behaviour, 21 January 2003. http://www.fhf.org.uk

11. C. Iribarren et al., 'Dietary Intake of Omega-3, Omega-6 Fatty Acids and Fish: Relationship With Hostility in Young Adults – The CARDIA Study', *European Journal of Clinical Nutrition* 2004, Vol. 58, No. 1.

12. D.S. Siscovick et al., 'Dietary Intake and Cell Membrane Levels of Long-Chain n-3 Polyunsaturated Fatty Acids and the Risk of Primary Cardiac Arrest', *Journal of the American Medical Association* 1995, Vol. 274 (17), pp. 1363–67.

13. A.P. Simopoulos and Jo Robinson, *The Omega Diet*, Harper Collins, 1999.

14. D.P. Rose et al., 'Influence of Diets Containing Eicosapentaenoic or Docosahexaenoic Acid on Growth and Metastasis of Breast Cancer Cells in Nude Mice', *Journal of the National Cancer Institute* 1995, Vol. 87 (8), pp. 587–92.

15. James Le Fanu, op. cit., pp. 348–9.

16. Sally Fallon and Mary G. Enig, 'It's the Beef – Myths and Truths About Beef', *Wise Traditions in Food, Farming and the Healing Arts*, Weston A. Price Foundation, Spring 2000.

Chapter 7

1. Colin Tudge, op. cit., p. 190.

2. Charles Darwin, *The Formation of Vegetable Mould Through the Action of Worms, with Observations on Their Habits*, John Murray, 1881, p. 148.

3. Elaine Ingham, 'The Soil Foodweb: Its Importance in Ecosystem

Health', A Report from the Department of Botany and Plant Pathology, Cordley Hall 2082, Oregon State University, Corvallis. http://www.soilfoodweb.com

4. David Pimental et al., 'Environmental, Energetic and Economic Comparisons of Organic and Conventional Farming', *Bioscience* July 2005, Vol. 55, No. 7, pp. 573–82.

5. The research results are summarized in John Reeves, *The Roots of Health*, available from Eastleigh, Greenfield Close, Joys Green, Lydbrook, Glos GL17 9RD, UK.

6. James Caird, *English Agriculture in 1850–51*, Frank Cass, Kelly Reprints of Economic Classics, 1967, pp. 457–8.

7. Tom Stockdale, 'Coronary Heart Disease – A New Perspective', *Nutrition and Health* 2004, Vol. 18, pp. 73–75.

Chapter 8

1. Uffe Ravnskov, *The Cholesterol Myths*, New Trends Publishing, Washington D.C., 2000.

2. James Le Fanu, *The Rise and Fall of Modern Medicine*, Abacus, 1999, p. 149.

3. Mary Enig, *Know Your Fats*, Bethesda Press, Silver Spring, 2000, cited in Ron Schmid, *The Untold Story of Milk,* New Trends Publishing, Washington D.C., 2003, p. 169.

4. Charles Sanford Porter, *Milk Diet as a Remedy for Chronic Disease*, Long Beach, California, 1905.

5. Sally Fallon, *Nourishing Traditions*, New Trends Publishing, Washington D.C., 1999, pp. 34–35.

6. J.R. Crewe, 'Raw Milk Cures Many Diseases', *Certified Milk Magazine* January 1929, pp. 3–6.

7. Jo Robinson, *Why Grassfed is Best*, Vashon Island Press, Vashon, Washington, 2000, p. 22.

8. T.R. Dhiman et al., 'Conjugated Linoleic Acid Content of Milk From Cows Fed Different Diets', *Journal of Dairy Science* 1999, Vol. 82 (10), pp. 2146–56.

9. H. Timmen and S. Patton, 'Milk Fat Globules: Fatty Acid Composition, Size and In Vivo Regulation of Fat Liquidity', *Lipids* 1988, Vol. 23, pp. 685–9.

10. Marius Collomb et al., 'Correlation Between Fatty Acids in Cows' Milk Produced in Lowlands, Mountains and Highlands of Switzerland and Botanical Composition of the Fodder', *International Dairy Journal* 2002, Vol. 12, pp. 661–8.

11. J.H. Nielsen and T. Lund-Nielsen, 'Healthier Organic Livestock Products: Antioxidants in Organic and Conventionally Produced Milk', *Book of Abstracts.* First Annual Congress of

the EU Project on Quality Low Input Food and the Soil Association Annual Conference, Newcastle 6–9 January 2005.

12. J. Robertson and C. Fanning. *Omega-3 Polyunsaturated Fatty Acids and Conventional Milk*, University of Aberdeen, 2004.

13. C.F. Garland et al., 'Can Colon Cancer Incidence and Death Rates be Reduced with Calcium and Vitamin D?' *American Journal of Clinical Nutrition* 1991, Vol. 54, p. 193S.

14. J.L. Outwater *et al.*, 'Dairy Products and Breast Cancer: The IGF-1, Oestrogen and bGH Hypothesis', *Medical Hypothesis* 1997, Vol. 48, pp. 453–61.

15. D.R. Davies, 'Healthier Organic Livestock Products: Avoiding Microbial Infections', *Book of Abstracts: Plenary Sessions and Technical Seminars*, 1st Annual Congree of the European Union Project on Quality Low Input Food and Soil Association Annual Conference, Newcastle, 6–9 January 2005.

16. Jonathan Long, 'Effective Control Strategy Keeps Mastitis Bills Down', *Farmers Weekly*, 21 October 2005.

17. Julian Mellentin, 'Omega Factor', Dairymen, Suppl. to *The Grocer*, 10 September 2005.

18. *Using Fatty Acids for Enhancing Classroom Achievement*, Report of Durham Educational Authority, January 2004. http://durhamtrial.org.uk

19. R.J. Dewhurst et al., 'Forage Breeding and Management to Increase the Beneficial Fatty Acid Content of Ruminant Products', *Proceedings of the Nutrition Society* 2003, Vol. 62, pp. 329–36.

20. Dairy Supply Chain Margins 2003–04, Milk Development Council, August 2004.

21. John Webster, 'More Respect, More Profit', *Farmers Weekly*, 28 October 2005.

22. A. J. Hosier, Open-Air Dairying, *Journal of the Farmers' Club*, Part 6, November 1927.

23. A Campaign for Real Milk. A Project of the Weston A. Price Foundation. http//www.realmilk.com

Chapter 9

1. Masanobu Fukuoka, *The One-Straw Revolution*, Other India Press, 1992, p. 2.

2. Department for Environment, Food and Rural Affairs, 2004 Harvest: Final Estimates of Cereal Production United Kingdom, 14 January 2005.

3. Masanobu Fukuoka, op. cit., pp. 65–6.

4. Newman Turner, *Fertility Farming*, Faber and Faber, 1951, pp. 17–18.
5. Department for Environment, Food and Rural Affairs, 'UK Farming in Context', Climate Change and Agriculture in the United Kingdom, 2000.
6. George Henderson, *The Farming Ladder*, Faber and Faber, 1944.
7. The present-day figure depends on the basis of the conversion. According to E.H. Net Economic History Services, using Gross Domestic Product as the basis of the conversion, the 2002 equivalent is around £497,000.
8. This is on the basis of the change in average earnings. See E.H. Net Economic History Services http://eh.net/hmit/ukcompare/
9. Colin Tudge, *So Shall We Reap*, Allen Lane, 2003, p. 83.
10. H.J. Massingham, *The Wisdom of the Fields*, Collins, 1945, p. 138.
11. *Feeding the Fifty Million*, A Report of the Rural Reconstruction Association Research Committee, Hollis and Carter, 1955, p. 95.
12. The estates were the Hiam Estate, a 7,000-acre holding in the Fens; Mr Rex Paterson's 11,000-acre estate in Hampshire; and Messrs. Parker's 30,000 acres in Norfolk, Lincolnshire and Leicestershire. The financial outputs of the three holdings were £220,600, £200,000 and £500,000, indicating a fall in output per acre as the size of holding increased. The figures were published in the 'Peterborough' column of the *Daily Telegraph*, on the 5 and 15 June 1943. George Henderson, op. cit., p. 166.
13. George Henderson, op. cit., p. 105.

Chapter 10

1. W.J. Reader, *Imperial Chemical Industries: A History, Vol. 1, 1870–1926*, Oxford University Press 1970.
2. Ibid. pp. 154–5.
3. W.J. Reader, *Imperial Chemical Industries: A History. Vol. 2. 1926–1952*, Oxford University Press, 1975.
4. Frederick Keeble, *Fertilizers and Food Production*, Oxford University Press, 1932, p. 61.
5. Philip Conford, 'A Forum for Organic Husbandry: The *New English Weekly* and Agricultural Policy, 1939–49', *Agricultural History Review* Vol. 46 (2), 1998, pp. 197–210.
6. Quentin Seddon, *The Silent Revolution*, BBC, pp. 21–22.
7. Colin Tudge, op. cit., p. 197.
8. H.J. Massingham (ed.), *England and the Farmer*, Batsford, 1941, p. 50.

9. OECD Paris, *Farm Household Income, Issues and Policy Responses*, 2003.
10. Colin Tudge, op. cit., p. 197.
11. Vaclav Smil, *Enriching the Earth*, MIT Press, 2001, pp. 155–76.

Chapter 11

1. The results were published in John Hamaker and Don Weaver's *The Survival of Civilization*, Hamaker-Weaver Publishers, Michigan, California, 1982. It is now published in a World Wide Web edition at: www.remineralize.org
2. John Hamaker, 'A Rock Dust Primer', *Remineralize the Earth*, Winter 1993–4, pp. 8–9.
3. Cameron Thomson, 'So what is rock dust and where do we get some', *Seer News*, Straloch Farm, Enochdhu, Blairgowrie, Winter 2002.
4. Julius Hensel, *Bread From Stones: A New and Rational System of Land Fertilization and Physical Regeneration*, 1892. The book is now published by Acres USA, P.O. Box 91299, Austin, Texas.
5. John David Mann, 'Bread From Stones', *Solstice*, May 1988, p. 51.
6. Bernard Jensen and Mark Anderson, *Empty Harvest*, Avery, 1990, p. 81.
7. Ibid.
8. Ocean Grown UK Ltd, P.O. Box 3833, Wincanton, BA9 8WY.
9. Maynard Murray, *Sea Energy Agriculture*, revised 2nd edn, Acres USA, 2003, p. 12.
10. Murray gives details of his trials in his book *Sea Energy Agriculture*. He records the location of the experiments, and where produce is analysed for particular nutrients, he records the testing laboratory.

Chapter 12

1. Colin Tudge, op. cit., p. 264.
2. Jules Pretty, 'The Real Costs of Modern Farming', *Resurgence*, March/April 2001.
3. Ibid.
4. 'Danish Pesticide Use Reduction Programme', Report of Pesticide Action Network Europe, June 2005.
5. J.N. Pretty et al., 'Farm Costs and Food Miles: An Assessment of the Full Cost of the UK Weekly Food Basket', *Food Policy* Vol. 30, No. 1, February 2005, pp. 1–19.

6. Alison Smith and Paul Watkiss, 'The Validity of Food Miles as an Indicator of Sustainable Development', Report for DEFRA by AEA Technology plc, July 2005.
7. Joanna Blythman, *Shopped – The Shocking Power of British Supermarkets*, Harper Perennial, 2004, p. 16.
8. *N. Pretty* et al., op. cit.

Chapter 13

1. Sally Fallon, *Nourishing Traditions*, New Trends Publishing, Washington DC, 1999, p. 34.
2. Edward Howell, *Enzyme Nutrition: The Food Enzyme Concept*, Avery, New York, 1985, pp. 100–1.
3. Peter King, *Traditional Cattle Breeds*, Farming Books and Videos, 2004, p. 17.
4. http://rbst.org.uk
5. Jim Worthington, *Natural Poultry-Keeping*, Crosby Lockwood, 1970.
6. Joel Salatin, 'Pastured Poultry: The Polyface Farm Model', The Weston A. Price Foundation, 11 August 2002, http://westonaprice.org
7. Sally Fallon, op. cit., p. 452.
8. Jen Allbritton, 'Wheaty Indiscretions', Weston A. Price Foundation, http://www.westonaprice.org
9. National Farmers' Retail and Markets Association, personal communication. http://www.farma.org.uk
10. 'Local Food Costs Less at Farmers' Markets', South West Local Food Partnership, March 2002.
11. http://www.seedsofhealth.co.uk
12. Charles Leigh, 'Food For Thought as Organic Sales Grow', *The Guardian*, 31 May 2005.

Appendix I

Name of mineral	Role in human health	Symptoms of deficiency
Calcium	Essential for normal function of the heart, blood clotting system and acid-alkaline balance. Promotes healthy skin, bone and teeth, plus normal nerve and muscular action.	Include muscle tremors, insomnia, nervousness, joint pain, high blood pressure and tooth decay.
Chromium	Essential for heart function and in the balancing of blood sugar. Helps protect DNA.	Sweating, hunger, drowsiness and thirst. Can lead to addiction to sweet foods.
Copper	Required for healthy growth and for liver, brain and muscle function. Also required for the regulation of blood cholesterol and for enzyme systems involved in antioxidant protection.	Conditions such as Crohn's or coeliac disease are associated with deficiency. Other symptoms include heart muscle weakness, anaemia, fluid retention and raised blood cholesterol. Excess levels can be toxic.
Iodine	Vital for the production of thyroid hormones, which control metabolic rate, conversion of food to energy and the maintenance of body temperature.	Include underactive or swollen thyroid gland, fatigue, weight gain, muscle weakness and susceptibility to cold.
Iron	As a component of haemoglobin, iron transports oxygen and carbon dioxide to and from cells. It is also essential for enzyme systems involved in energy production.	Include anaemia, fatigue, listlessness, poor appetite and nausea.

Name of mineral	Role in human health	Symptoms of deficiency
Magnesium	Strengthens bones and teeth and aids muscle function. Required for cardiac and nervous systems. Important for energy production and many enzyme systems.	Muscle spasms, insomnia, nervousness, high blood pressure, heart palpitations, hyperactivity, depression and fits.
Manganese	Aids in the formation of bones, cartilage and nerve tissue. Vital to a number of enzyme systems including those conferring immunity. Also stabilizes blood sugar, promotes healthy DNA, aids reproduction and red blood cell synthesis. Required for brain function and insulin production.	Muscle twitching, growing pains in children, dizziness, fits and joint pain.
Molybdenum	Aids the removal of protein breakdown products, and strengthens teeth. Helps detoxify the body of free radicals.	Deficiency symptoms rarely seen except where copper or sulphate interfere with its utilization. They may include anaemia, tooth decay, impotence, irregular pulse and hyperventilation.
Phosphorus	A structural component of bones and teeth. Vital to normal metabolism, energy production and acidity regulation. Required for optimum athletic performance.	Unlikely to be deficient because it is present in most foods. Signs of deficiency can include loss of appetite, susceptibility to infection, anaemia, muscle weakness, bone and joint pain, nervous system changes.
Potassium	Aids the flow of nutrients between cells, promotes healthy muscles and nerves. Important for insulin secretion and normal metabolism. Maintains heart function and gut movement.	Include irregular heartbeat, muscle weakness, pins and needles, nausea, vomiting, diarrhoea and low blood pressure.
Selenium	An important antioxidant, selenium is required for efficient immune function and protection against cancer and infections. Also important for normal cell growth and the regulation of thyroid hormone production.	Low selenium intakes greatly increase the risk of many cancers. Deficiency is also associated with premature ageing, cataracts, high blood pressure and frequent infections.
Sodium	Maintains the body's water balance. Aids nerve function and muscle action, as well as helping move nutrients into cells.	Include dizziness, heat exhaustion, low blood pressure, mental apathy, muscle cramps, nausea, vomiting and headache.

Name of mineral	Role in human health	Symptoms of deficiency
Zinc	A component of many enzyme systems as well as DNA and RNA. Vital for growth and healing. Controls hormones and promotes brain function and a healthy nervous system. Aids bone and teeth formation.	Include diminished sense of smell and taste, frequent infections, acne, low fertility, skin pallor, depression and appetite loss.

Sources: Patrick Holford, *New Optimum Nutrition Bible*, Piatkus, 2004; Dr Sarah Brewer, *The Daily Telegraph Encyclopedia of Vitamins, Minerals and Herbal Supplements*, Constable & Robinson, 2002.

Index